Heaven Scent

AROMATIC CHRISTMAS CRAFTS, RECIPES, and DECORATIONS

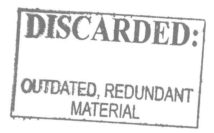

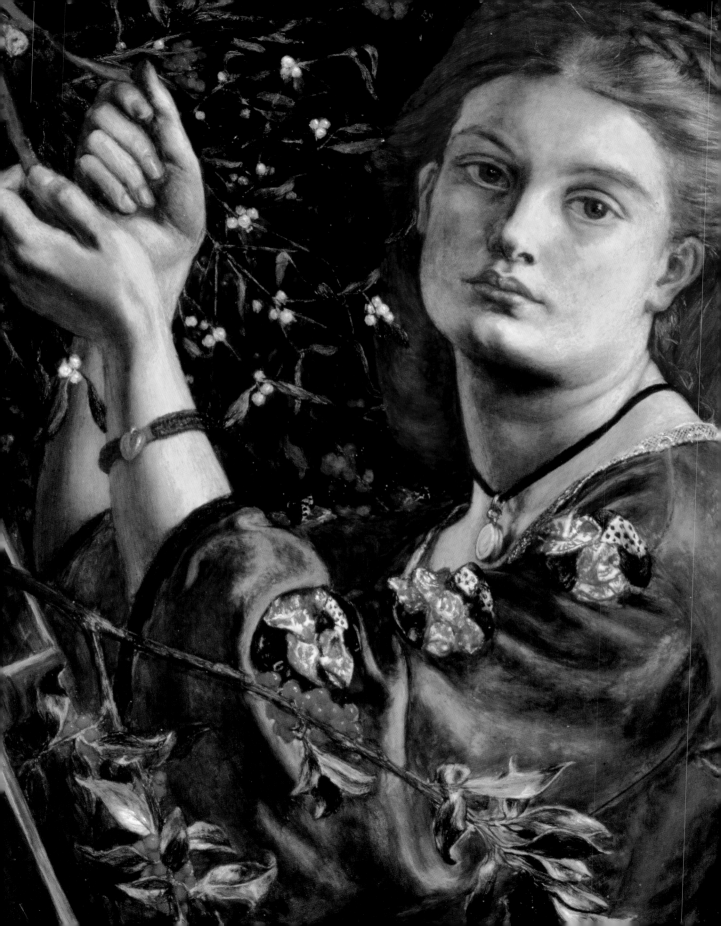

JULIA LAWLESS

Heaven Scent

AROMATIC CHRISTMAS CRAFTS, RECIPES, *and* DECORATIONS

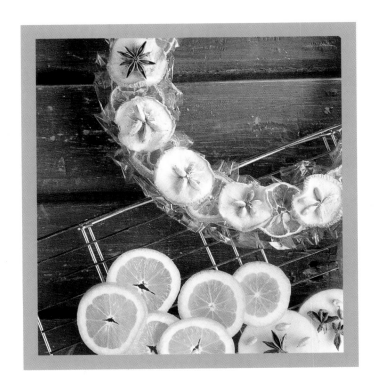

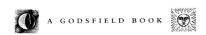 A GODSFIELD BOOK

Library of Congress Cataloging-in-Publication Data Available

10 9 8 7 6 5 4 3 2 1

Published in 1998 by Sterling Publishing Company, Inc.
387 Park Avenue South, New York, N.Y. 10016

Produced for Sterling Publishing by
Godsfield Press Limited

Designed by
The Bridgewater Book Company Ltd.

Picture Research *Vanessa Fletcher*
Studio Photography *Paul Forrester*
Stylist *Pamela Westland*

Distributed in Canada by Sterling Publishing
c/o Canadian Manda Group, One Atlantic Avenue, Suite 105
Toronto, Ontario, Canada M6K 3E7
Distributed in Australia by Capricorn Link (Australia) Pty Ltd
P. O. Box 6651, Baulkham Hills, Business Centre, NSW 2153, Australia

Printed and bound in Hong Kong

ISBN 0-8069-7062-6

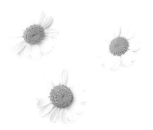

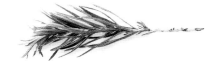

Contents

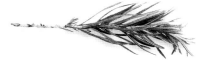

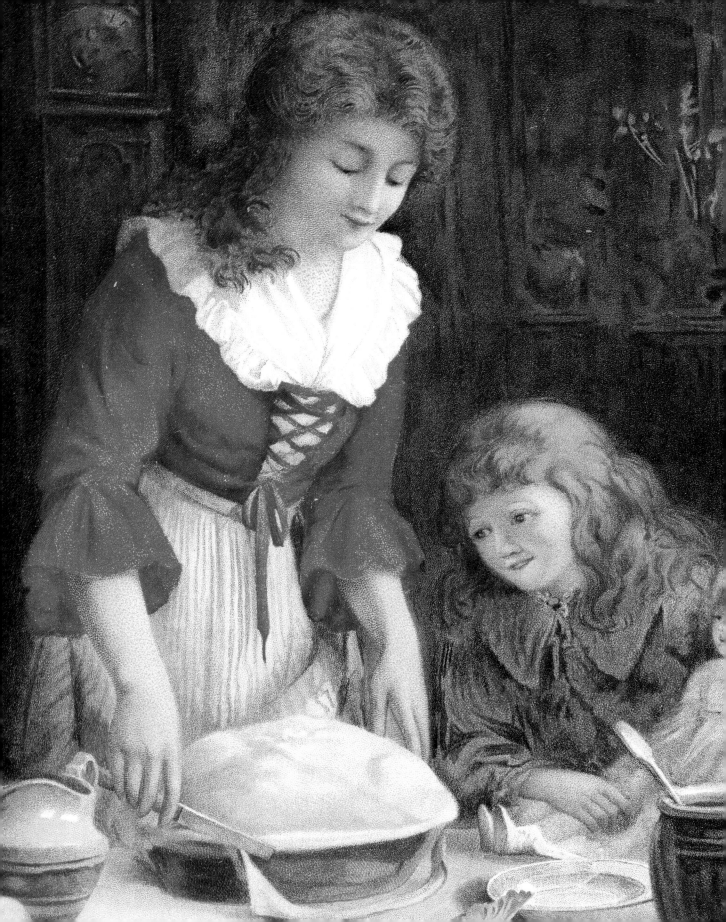

INTRODUCTION

The Symbolism of Christmas

HERBS, SPICES, AND PERFUMES have always played a major role in Christmas celebrations. The power of fragrance is well known for its ability to stir the imagination and recall forgotten memories. Perfumes such as frankincense, myrrh, clove, and cinnamon can conjure up a kaleidoscope of imagery, the magic of the East, the ancient spice trail.

Many traditional foods, such as mince pies, plum pudding, and Christmas cake, are richly flavored with spices and candied fruit. The Christmas tree has a pleasing smell, reminiscent of northern pine woods, and it is customary to make and burn scented candles. When all these aromatic scents mingle together, they not only create a homely feeling of warmth and comfort, but also help to evoke a festive atmosphere.

"At the Winter Solstice, the Great Mother, Queen of Heaven, gives birth to the Son of Light... it symbolizes ascent and the growing power of the sun."

ADVENT

Advent (from the Latin "to come") begins on the fourth Sunday before Christmas. Special Advent decorations can provide a symbolic centerpiece in the home during this period. These may be wreaths woven from fir twigs, or a table arrangement of four candles surrounded by sprays of evergreens, pine cones and flowers. It is customary to light one candle on each of the four Sundays of Advent. When

LEFT: Puddings and pies complete the kitchen table.

RIGHT: Pumpkin and squash produce rich aromas when cooking.

all four candles are lit on the final Sunday, completing the wreath or crown, they herald the birth of Christ.

Scandinavian, Dutch, and German families bake an assortment of spicy, decorative cookies for Advent, particularly on December 6th, the feast of St. Nicholas.

WINTER FESTIVALS

Christmas and Easter are the two most important events in the Christian calendar, yet many of their accompanying rituals can be traced to a time before Christianity.

✳ ROMAN ORIGINS – The tradition of feasting, playing games, and performing pantomimes originates in the midwinter festivities of the Romans, particularly the festival

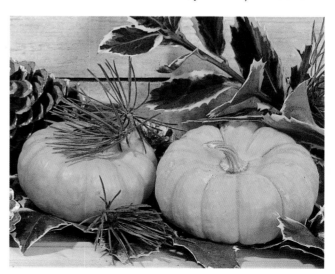

of Saturnalia on December 17th. At this great festival, everything was turned upside-down: masters waited on their servants, gambling and drunkenness were encouraged, men dressed as women, and women posed as men!

Evergreen trees were also decorated at this time of year and sometimes brought into the house, while gifts were exchanged at Kalends, the Roman New Year. In Scotland, it is still customary to give gifts at New Year (Hogmanay), and for friends and family to hold hands in a circle and sing "Auld Lang Syne"– a song based on the belief that ancestors return to the family hearth at the turn of the year.

"The holly and the ivy, when
they are both full grown
Of all the trees that are in the wood,
the holly bears the crown."
TRADITIONAL CHRISTMAS CAROL

✶ WINTER SOLSTICE – December 21st marks the ancient pagan celebration of the winter solstice: the shortest day of the year, after which the days begin to lengthen and the dormant forces of nature start to stir once again.

The ancient Persian festival of Mithras, "the day of the birth of the unconquered sun," also fell in late December. Thus, alongside its religious values, the midwinter festival of Christmas assimilated ancient pagan beliefs where the cycles of nature and the changing seasons were revered with special ceremonies.

✶ HANUKKAH – Hanukkah, the Jewish festival of lights, which commemorates the rededication of the temple by Judas Maccabaeus in 165 B.C., falls in late November or December. Children receive presents, and a candle is lit each night on a branched candelabrum, called a menorah.

✶ ST LUCIA – The Feast of St. Lucia, which falls on December 13th, marks the beginning of the Christmas season in many Scandinavian countries. A "Lucia Procession" is still common in Sweden today. A young girl, dressed in a white gown (representing light) and a red sash (symbolizing fire), wearing a crown of woven bilberry twigs with nine lighted candles, parades through the village. She visits each house in turn, bringing them her blessing. She is accompanied by a company of trolls, representing the darker aspects of nature.

CHRISTMAS EVE

Traditionally, Christmas Eve was the time when the house was decorated and celebrations began in earnest. The custom of decking the home with holly, ivy, mistletoe, and other fresh-scented evergreens harks back to a time when many plants held a special significance.

Both the holly and ivy have been credited with protective powers, especially potent in the dead of winter. When brought indoors, these plants would protect the household from all sorts of disturbances over the holy season — especially lightning, witchcraft, and goblins! Later, within the Christian tradition, the holly's prickly leaves became associated with the crown of thorns and the red berries with drops of Christ's blood.

The introduction of the Christmas tree as a central festive symbol is relatively modern, only becoming popular in the late nineteenth century (it was introduced to England by Queen Victoria's husband, Albert). As an evergreen, the fir tree (like the tree of life in the Bible) represents the unchanging or immortal status of the soul.

CHRISTMAS FOOD

Christmas, of course, is also a feast day! For a medieval lord, a boar's head garnished with bay and rosemary would have dominated the table. Later, a roast goose stuffed with sage and onions became the traditional Christmas meal. Nowadays turkey, which lends itself to a variety of aromatic flavors and combinations, is the most popular Christmas dish in England. In the USA, where turkey is more usually eaten at Thanksgiving, ham often takes pride of place on the Christmas table.

RIGHT: Christmas acquired most of its familiar trappings during the nineteenth century.

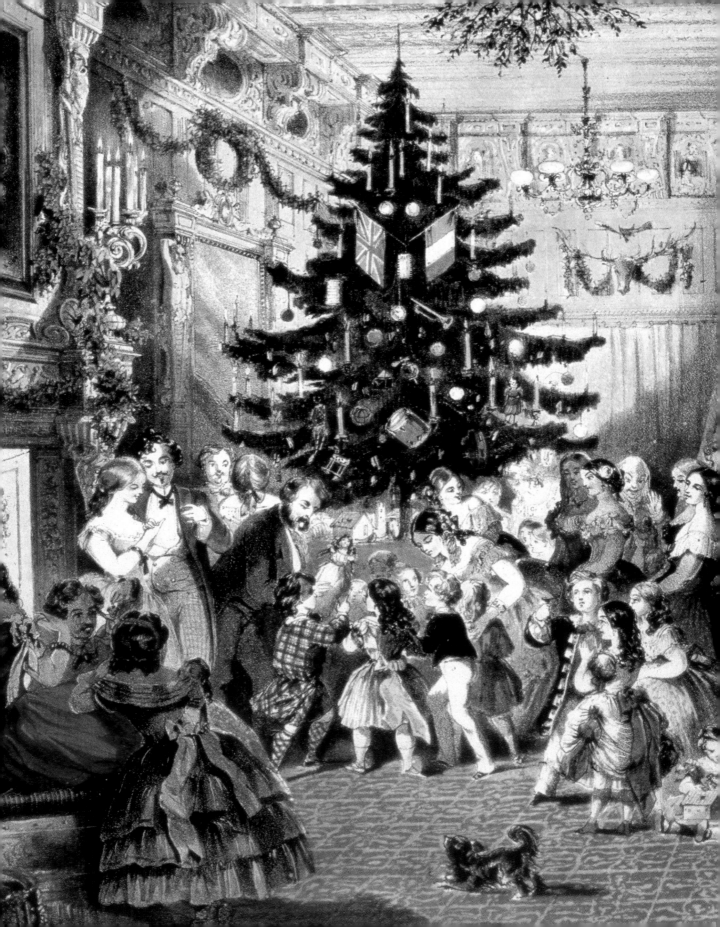

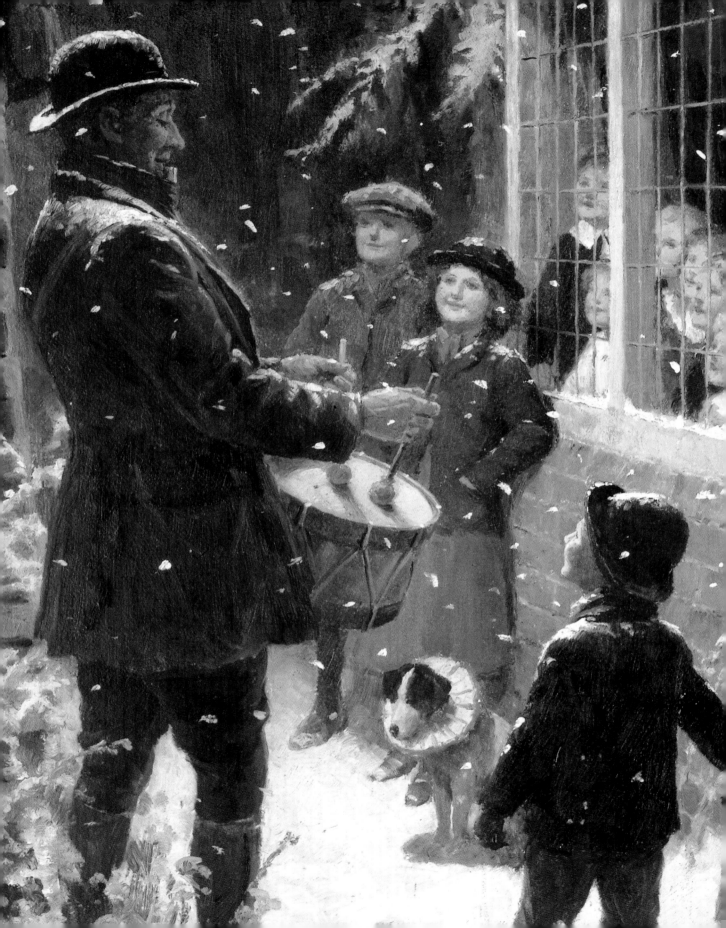

NEW YEAR

New Year's Eve has always been celebrated with late-night revelry. Family and friends traditionally shared a bowl of spiced ale and stayed up until midnight to see the New Year in. The head of the family would drink first, offering a toast of "Wassail" (meaning "Good health"), and then the bowl would be passed around.

LEFT: Bringing music to the neighborhood is part of tradition.

The first man to cross the threshold after midnight was known as the "lucky bird," or "first foot." He would bring with him offerings of bread, salt, and coal – the symbols of life, hospitality, and warmth.

It was a time to look back on the achievements and failures of the past year and to make fresh resolutions for the coming year. In parts of Scotland it was traditional to clean and polish the whole house, mend any torn clothes, change all the beds and generally make ready for the New Year. Songs would be sung and poems recited in a spirit of merriment; sometimes groups of people would go from house to house doing this.

GOLD, FRANKINCENSE, AND MYRRH

Originally, the "holy season" was considered to begin on the night of Christmas Eve and continue until Epiphany on January 6th. This is when the Magi are said to have brought their gifts of gold, frankincense, and myrrh to the baby Jesus – the symbols of kingship, divinity, and passion.

During Christ's lifetime, frankincense played a central role in many religious ceremonies, both as an offering and as a means of communication with the divine. It was so important that a special frankincense route was developed by Arabian traders to assist with its distribution, its high value being matched only by myrrh and gold.

Myrrh gets its name from the Arabic word *murr,* meaning "bitter," because of its bitter taste. Myrrh was also used as incense and respected throughout the ancient world as a medicine and purifying agent.

TWELFTH NIGHT

Twelve days after Christmas, decorations are taken down, marking the end of the holy season. Traditionally, a special cake was eaten on this occasion: Twelfth Night cake or, as the French still call it, *galette des rois.* A treasure, such as a coin, would be concealed inside it; or alternatively a dried pea and a dried bean. The person who found the bean was King for the night; the person who found the pea was Queen.

Twelfth Night cake began to go out of fashion in the 1850s, its place usurped by the Christmas pudding, served complete with silver sixpences, dried fruits, a sprig of holly and a splash of brandy.

"Wassail wassail all over the town, our toast it is white and our ale it is brown, our bowl it is made of the white maple tree, with the wassailing bowl we drink to thee."

TRADITIONAL GLOUCESTERSHIRE WASSAIL SONG
Festivals, Family and Food, D. Carey and J. Large.

CELEBRATE!

The traditions and rituals associated with Christmas – feasting and drinking, lighting candles, burning sweet-scented logs, exchanging gifts and enjoying good company amidst the rich aromas of incense and spices in a warm, convivial atmosphere – are all inherent and time-honored aspects of this festive season.

The financial cost of Christmas can be a burden to many families. However, presents do not need to be costly or extravagant. Celebrate your creative spirit by making your own cards, decorations, and individually designed presents: it is very satisfying. Everyone loves to receive a handmade gift. This book will give you lots of ideas for attractive, "heaven scent" aromatic decorations and gifts. It may also spark you off on some new creative paths of your own!

AROMATIC OILS AND SPICES

Christmas Oils and Spices

BAY

The fresh, spicy-scented leaves of this handsome evergreen shrub have been used for making garlands since ancient times. To the Romans, the bay was a symbol of renewal, and they were probably the first to hang a wreath of bay leaves on their doors at New Year to bring good luck.

Bay is well known for its culinary uses and as an ingredient in bouquet garni. Fresh bay leaves are great for making all kinds of household decorations at Christmas. The oil can be used in pot-pourri, and for making linen bags, as it helps to keep insects away from cloth.

FRANKINCENSE

Frankincense is an aromatic resin which exudes from the bark of a small tree, native to the desert regions of the Red Sea. Civilizations of both the East and West made use of frankincense for religious rituals and ceremonies, and of course it was given to the Christ-child by the Magi. Complete cities were built on the wealth derived from the trade in this precious substance in the ancient world.

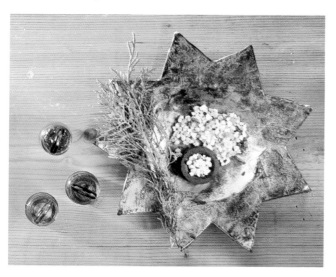

Oil of frankincense (as grains or sticks) can be burned as an incense at home over the Christmas period. Frankincense oil can also be added to massage or bath oils for its restorative qualities, and makes an excellent long-lasting fixative for pot-pourri blends.

LAVENDER

Lavender is probably the most popular of all the scented herbs and plants. Because the leaves and flowers retain their scent and color so well after drying, it has traditionally been used for creating all kinds of winter and Christmas decorations, such as herb posies, garlands, and topiary. It can be used to make a wide range of Christmas gifts such as linen bags, pot-pourri, herb pillows, and bath sacs.

The oil makes a relaxing room fragrance and can also be used to revive pot-pourri or scent items such as writing paper, ink, and cloth. For hundreds of years, it has been an essential ingredient in preparations such as eau-de-cologne, flower waters, soaps, and bath oils.

MYRRH

Like frankincense, myrrh is a natural gum resin derived from the bark of a small tree which is found in the arid areas of north-east Africa and the Red Sea region. It has been used as an incense, perfume, and medicinal agent for over 3,700 years.

Myrrh oil is a pale yellow liquid which is healing, soothing, and purifying. It has a slightly sharp, balsamic scent which combines well with spice oils, frankincense, and orange, when burned as a room fragrance. Its perfume is very rich and long-lasting, which makes it a valuable ingredient in pot-pourri blends and for fixing or stabilizing more volatile scents such as orange or pine.

LEFT: A one-off dish makes an excellent display container.

RIGHT: Personalize pot-pourri with a favorite blend of spices.

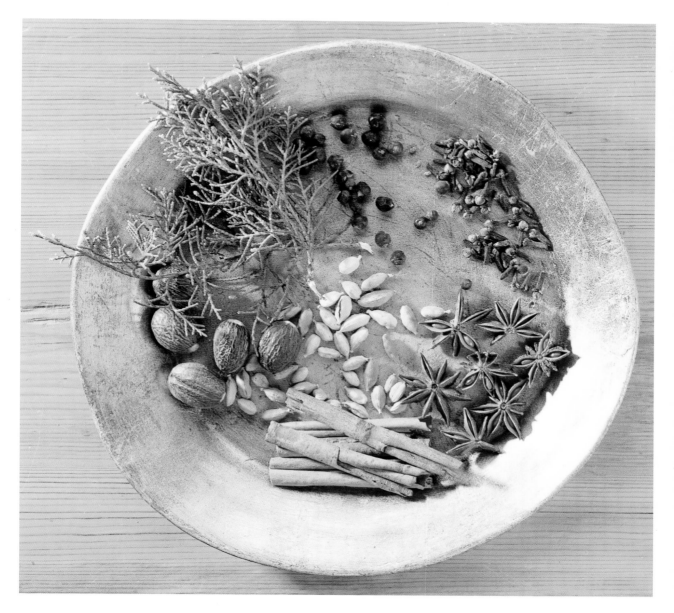

ORANGE

Orange oil is obtained from the peel of the fruit, where it is so plentiful that it actually squirts out if you squeeze it! The fresh, tangy scent of orange pomanders has traditionally been used at Christmas to help create a warm, festive atmosphere. Symbolically, the orange is associated with the sun and the return of lighter days after the winter solstice.

Oranges, mandarins, and kumquats make colorful Christmas decorations, combined with greenery. Dried orange peel and orange oil can be used in pot-pourri. Orange oil makes an uplifting room fragrance, and children especially are fond of its familar sweet fragrance.

PINE

Pine and fir trees have become central symbols of Christmas. The tradition of bringing a "Christmas tree" indoors is of German origin, although the custom of decorating the house with evergreen branches over the winter months can be traced back to pagan times. Fresh sprays of pine, larch, fir or juniper can be used to make all kinds of decorations including swags, wreaths and garlands.

Pine oil, which has a characteristic fresh, balsamic scent, is made from the needles of the tree. It makes an invigorating room fragrance or bath oil. It can be used to revive pot-pourri and to scent pine cones.

CARDAMOM

This spice has been used since the earliest times as a medicine, for flavoring food, and as an incense. Known in Europe as the "Fire of Venus," it was also used in medieval love potions because of its reputed aphrodisiac properties! In Victorian England, the seeds were chewed to sweeten the breath after meals.

Cardamom is good for flavoring all kinds of pickles, fruit compôtes, mulled wines, and spicy festive dishes. Store the seeds whole, as their flavor deteriorates rapidly once they are ground. The seeds and oil can be used in pot-pourri and herb sachets. It has a very strong smell and tends to overshadow other scents.

CINNAMON

Cinnamon was one of the most valuable spices of the ancient world, where it was used as a medicine, an incense and a perfume material. Like cardamom, it was also once considered to be a potent aphrodisiac. It was an essential ingredient in medieval cooking, particularly in France. Today it is used in puddings, fruit-based dishes, meat, pickles, mulled wine and spiced ales.

Bind cinnamon sticks with ribbon to make aromatic Christmas decorations. The bark (or oil) also makes an attractive addition to pot-pourri blends; added to linen sachets, it helps to repel moths.

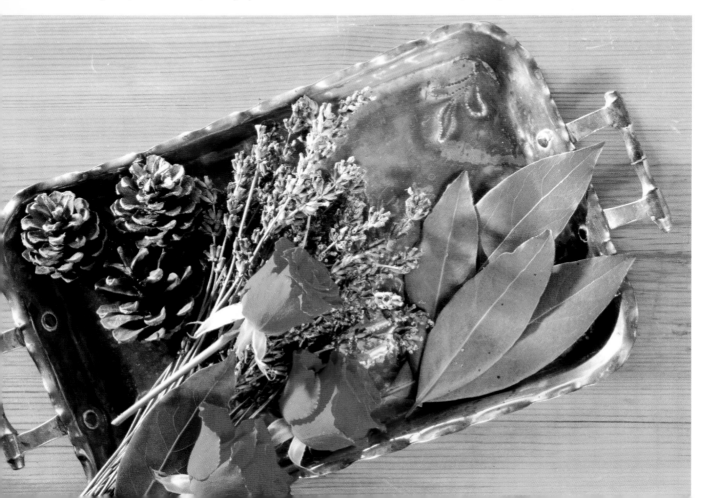

CLOVES

At one time, clove buds were chewed to sweeten the breath and were considered to be a panacea for all kinds of illness. Clove oil is a good treatment for toothache. In the Middle Ages, oranges stuck with cloves, called pomanders, were used to help keep disease at bay.

Cloves, like cinnamon and cardamom, are better stored whole to preserve potency, and are frequently used in the same recipes. At Christmas, cloves are especially valuable for flavoring ham, wine, fruit preserves, pickles, and cooked apples. Use the whole clove buds (or oil) in pot-pourri, linen sachets, and for making pomanders.

GINGER

Warming and rich, the root of the ginger plant has been used as a perfume, remedy, and culinary spice for thousands of years. In India and China it is known as a "universal medicine" because it has so many uses, being especially valuable during the winter months. It is also a powerful stimulant and tonic, and said to be an aphrodisiac.

LEFT: Bay, lavender, and pine cones all leave a lingering fragrance.

RIGHT: Dried fruit and ginger have spicy, warm scents.

Dried ginger is hotter than the fresh root, and is used for different purposes: powdered ginger is more suitable for cakes and confectionery, while the fresh root is better for pickles and savory meat or fish dishes. Crystallized ginger root also makes an exotic after-dinner sweet and breath freshener.

JUNIPER

Juniper berries have been used for cookery, in medicines, and for perfumery since ancient times. Sprigs of juniper were used as incense by early civilizations, including the Romans and Greeks. Juniper berries are commonly used in eastern European dishes; they also feature in traditional Christmas recipes such as salt beef and red cabbage.

Evergreen sprays of fresh juniper, with their fresh, tangy scent, are great for making all kinds of Christmas decorations. The berries are useful for flavoring food and

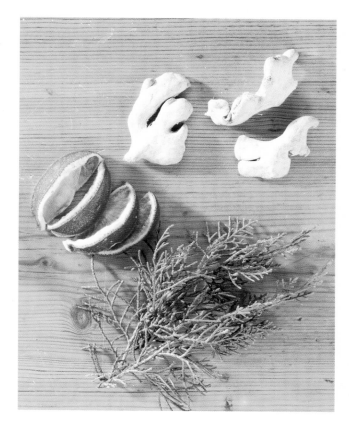

drinks (especially gin) and for adding to pot-pourri. Juniper oil can be used in in bath preparations, toiletries, and as an aromatic incense.

NUTMEG

An exotic spice, nutmeg was originally used as a medicine. In small quantities, it was used to aid digestion; in larger amounts it was well known for its narcotic effects. As a culinary spice it adds richness and warmth to all kinds of festive dishes, mulled wine or ale. It has long been used to flavor cakes and puddings. Nutmeg is best stored whole in airtight containers, as it loses its sweet-smelling qualities quickly once ground.

Whole nutmegs can be used to decorative effect in Christmas decorations such as swags and garlands. The powdered spice and oil can also be used in pot-pourri and herb sachets.

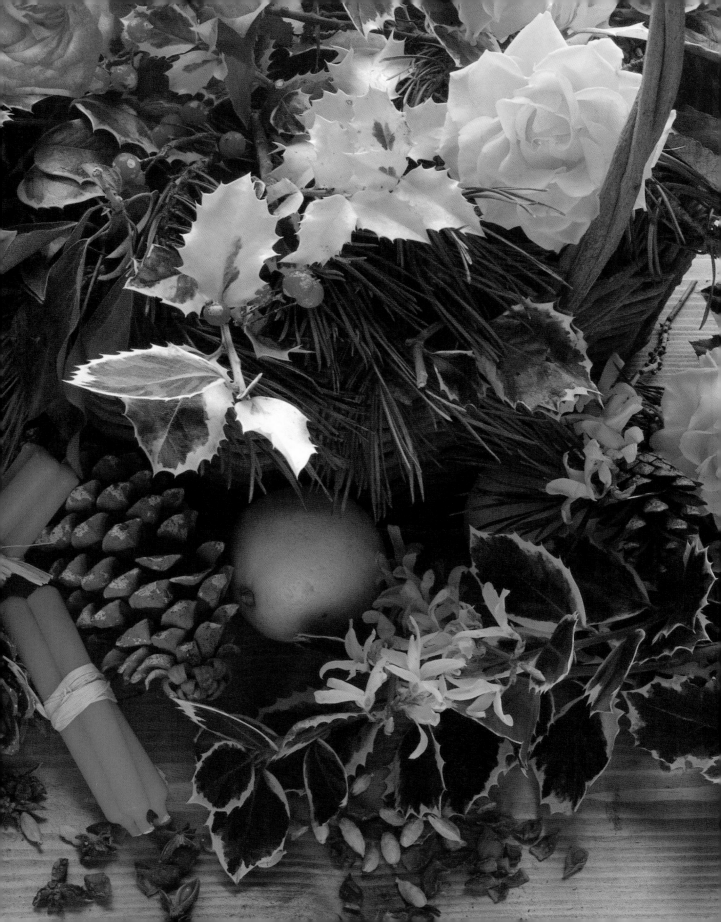

PART ONE

Christmas Decorations

THE CUSTOM OF DECORATING *the home with greenery during the cold winter months is a long established tradition. Its origins stretch back deep into a time before Christianity and the celebration of Christmas, to pagan festivals where people looked forward to the return of the sun at the darkest point in the year.*

Many of the decorative ideas outlined on the following pages reflect the individual ways in which different cultures have, over the centuries, captured the spirit of the season. Candles, dried fruits and evergreens, together with the rich, aromatic qualities of herbs and flowers dried or preserved during the summer months, have always played a central role at Christmas time and been used to brighten the home in the bleak season of winter.

"With spangles gay and candle light
And many toys, our tree is bright
And gold and silver birds are there:
While over all there hangs a star."

At one time, many country houses had a still room where plants were prepared and stored. Flower waters and perfumes were mixed, and aromatic remedies were concocted according to household recipes. You may not have the luxury of a special room to work on these crafts, but the projects can just as easily be carried out on the kitchen table or in a garden shed.

If it is not practical to gather plant materials directly from your garden or

LEFT: Dried flowers give a hint of spring in the depths of winter.

RIGHT: You can use fruits and nuts to decorate your table.

from the countryside, then most of the items mentioned in this book are readily available from florists' shops. Save the petals from shop-bought cut flowers and dry them for later use in a pot-pourri.

When making your decorations, a large part of the enjoyment is in the challenge of creating an individual design using materials which are to hand — therefore, although the following suggestions provide a rough framework of ideas as a guideline, allow your imagination a free rein!

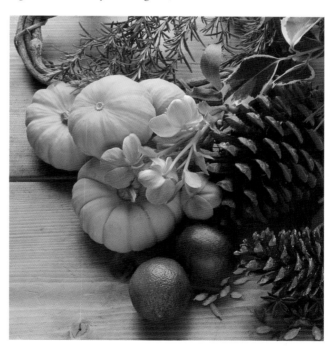

A Welcoming Garland

ONE ANCIENT CUSTOM, still very much alive today, is that of hanging a welcoming garland of evergreens on the front door of your house at the beginning of the Christmas season. Today's garlands are made from all manner of evergreen leaves including holly, ivy, yew, cherry laurel and spruce, but in the past they were always constructed entirely from bay laurel.

The bay tree has a rich symbolic history. In ancient Greece, bay leaves represented courage, while to the Romans, bay was also a symbol of renewal or eternal life, because its leaves did not fall or wither. The Romans hung a wreath of bay leaves on the door at New Year to bring good luck. Later, bay was ascribed with protective powers, probably due to its excellent

---

YOU WILL NEED

Evergreens: short sprays of cypress (with mini brown cones), variegated holly with red berries, viburnum or bay laurel leaves, blue pine

Double wire ring (from florist's)

Dry moss, Pine cones, Floristry wire

Floristry stub wires, Green twine

Decorative ribbons (optional)

METHOD

✳ Bend the wire ring into a heart-shaped frame. Cover the frame with moss, using green twine to bind it on.

✳ Make up small bunches of each type of evergreen, binding them with wire. Using wire, attach the bunches to the base one by one, overlapping them so that the leaves conceal the binding wire of the previous bunch. Work your way round the frame. Twist the pine cones on to stub wires, and fix to the frame.

✳ Attach green twine or wire to the frame to hang it with.

✳ Spray the wreath with water daily, to keep it looking fresh.

antiseptic qualities, and in the Middle Ages it was hung at the entrance of a house in the belief that it warded off evil: "Neither witch nor devil, thunder nor lightning, will hurt a man where a bay tree is."

A bay tree, planted in a tub beside the front door of a house, is still a familiar sight, although the symbolic associations may have been forgotten.

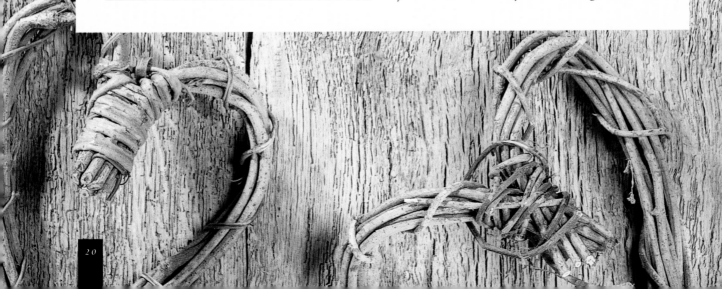

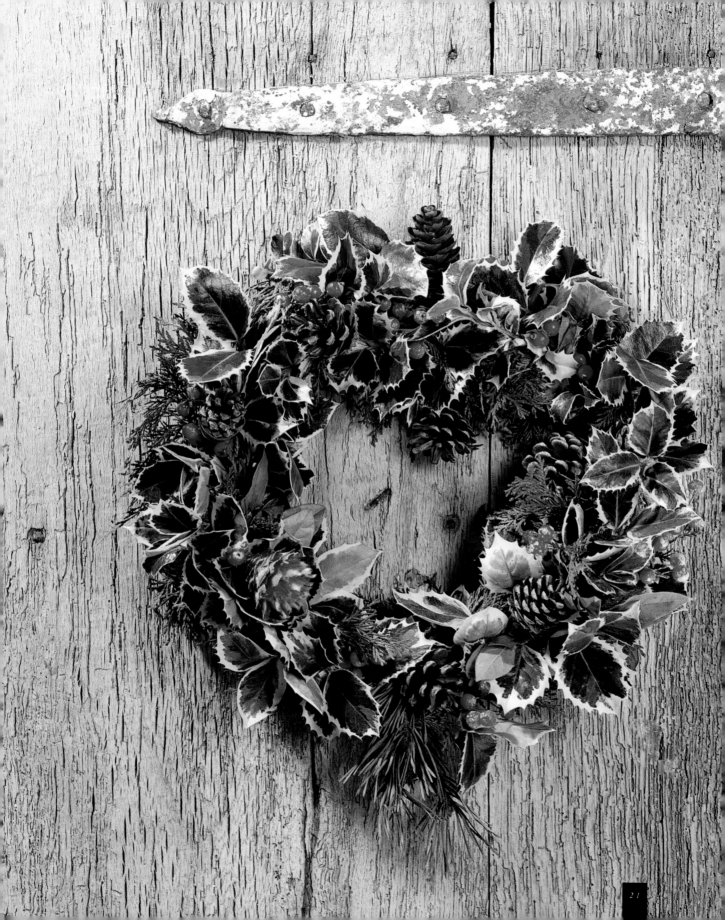

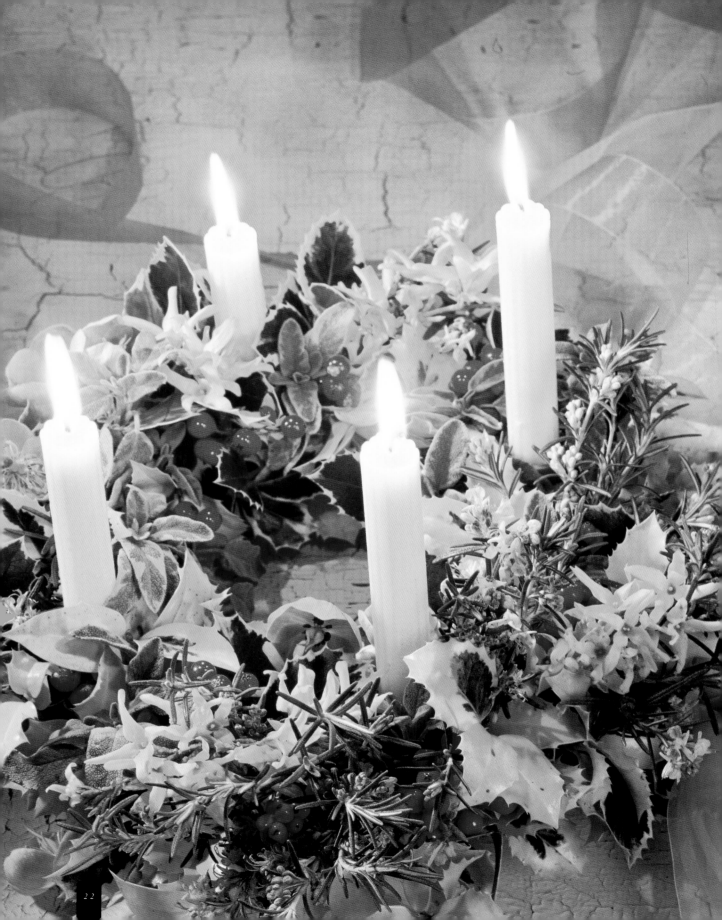

An Advent Centerpiece

THE COUNTDOWN TO CHRISTMAS day begins one month beforehand, with the four weeks of Advent (from the Latin words meaning "to come"). In many countries, the Advent period is traditionally celebrated both at home and in places of worship by the lighting of a candle on each successive Sunday preceding Christmas.

A candlelit circlet constructed from evergreen leaves, fresh flowers and ribbons provides an attractive, symbolic focal point in the home throughout the busy period leading up to Christmas. Our Advent centrepiece is a delicate arrangement based on a gold, green and cream colour scheme — but a combination of bright reds and golds can be just as effective.

YOU WILL NEED

8in (20cm) floristry foam ring (or Oasis)

4 cream candles, 4 plastic candle spikes

Short sprays of evergreens: variegated holly with red berries, variegated sage, rosemary

Fresh flowers: green hellebores (*Helleborus orientalis*), winter jasmine

1yd (1m) each of 1½in (4cm) wide sheer ribbon in cream, pale green, pale yellow

1 floristry stub wire

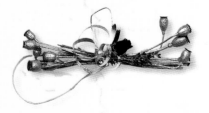

METHOD

✳ Soak the foam ring in water. Insert the candle spikes into the ring and press the candles firmly into them, making sure they are secure.

✳ Create a dense foliage background by pushing the holly and sage into the foam, making sure that the candles are not touching any of the leaves.

✳ Add clusters of rosemary and winter jasmine. Gently insert the hellebores at intervals.

✳ Finally, to provide the finishing touch, twist the ribbons into a bow. Thread the stub wire through the base of the bow and push it into the foam.

✳ Place the ring in the centre of a shallow bowl or dish filled with water, which could in turn be concealed within a low basket if desired. Check water levels daily, and top up with fresh water as required. Kept in a cool room, this arrangement should last for the whole of the Advent period.

✳ Never leave burning candles unattended.

✳ As an innovative alternative arrangement, simply put four floating candles in an attractive shallow bowl filled with water. Float other decorative items alongside. Children will enjoy choosing different flower heads, leaves or other colorful items such as gilded fir cones to float on the surface. To enhance the fragrance, add a few drops of selected essential oils to the water.

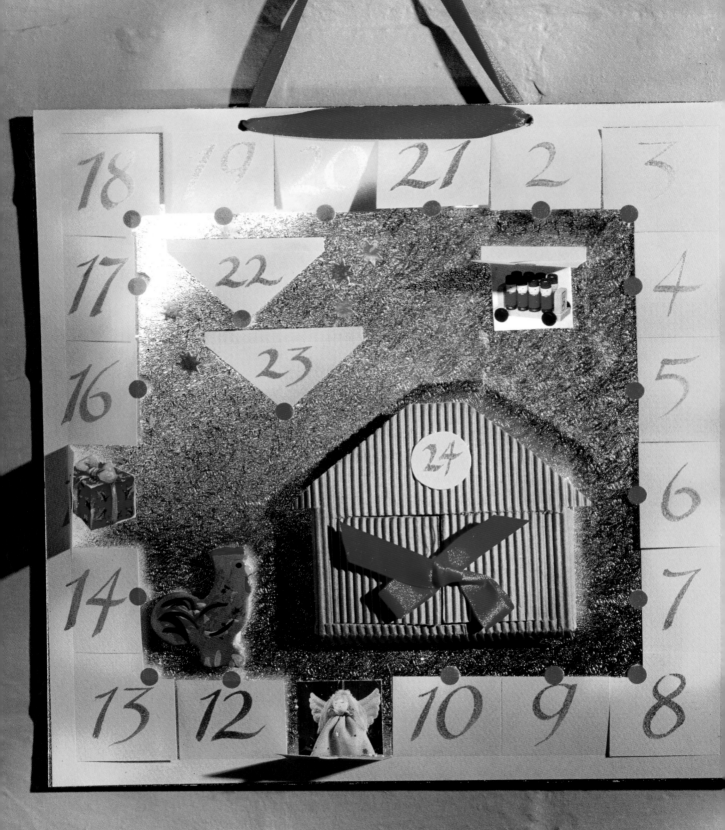

Aromatic Advent Calendar

ADVENT IS a time of preparation, when children can busy themselves making cards, decorations, gifts and sweets in readiness for the festive season. Focus the excitement of looking forward to Christmas Day with an Advent calendar. Traditionally, this can either take the form of a paper picture with opening windows, or a string of tiny presents, such as nuts, sweets, or marbles — one for each day of December up to Christmas Eve.

YOU WILL NEED

Cake board, Large empty matchbox

Corrugated card, Glue

Red ribbon, Nativity cake decoration

Old Christmas cards, Yellow card

Red sticky paper dots

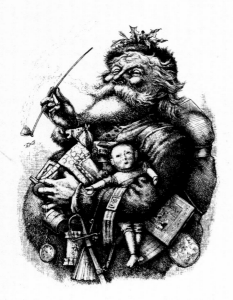

METHOD

✻ *Use the cake board as a base for the Advent calendar. Take the empty matchbox and cover it with corrugated card, using an extended piece at the front for a roof shape. Glue in place. Cut two big doors in the front. Fix a piece of ribbon to each door to close it with. Put the Nativity cake decoration inside the matchbox. (Or make your own figures out of marzipan.) Tie the doors together with a bow.*

✻ *Make the pictures to place behind the rest of the Advent doors, by cutting out appropriate images from Christmas cards. Glue these round the edge of the cake board.*

✻ *Make the doors. Cut a piece of yellow card the same size as the cake board. Cut a square out of the center, leaving a big enough piece round the edge to form the doors. Score a narrow strip all the way round the square, ½in (1cm) from the edge. Cut the doors, snipping as far as the scored strip. Bend back the doors. Glue the piece to the cake board along the narrow strip. Use the sticky red dots to close the yellow doors.*

✻ *Add extra doors (and Christmas images) to the center of the cake board. Make sure that you have a total of 24 doors, including the matchbox.*

✻ *Write the numbers on the doors. Punch two holes in the board and hang the calendar with red ribbon.*

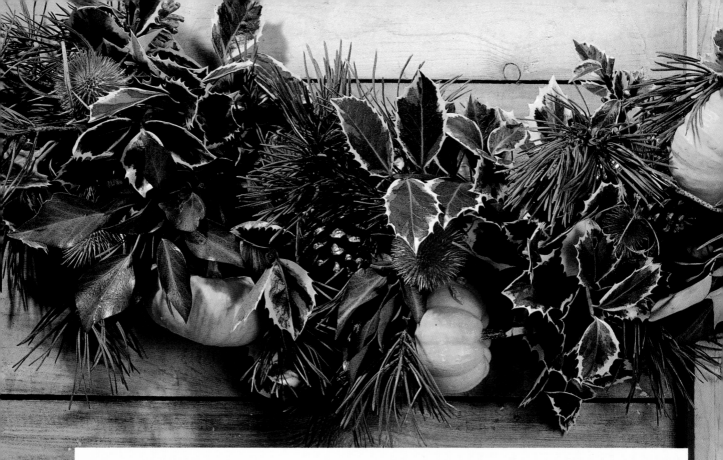

An Evergreen Garland

A LONG, ELABORATE GARLAND constructed from aromatic plant materials makes a spectacular decorative feature for Thanksgiving or Christmas. It can be displayed over a door or mirror, hung above a fireplace, draped along a beam, looped around banisters, or even placed to snake down the center of the dining table.

Our garland is made from a mixture of fresh and dried materials, but it is possible to construct the chain from any combination of evergreens, dried plant materials, seedheads, bunches of spices, dried fruit, ribbons, or other decorations. Gilding various items adds an extra festive gleam. Traditionally, plants such as holly, ivy, and misletoe were regarded as particularly powerful life-giving symbols because they remain green and bear their berries in the depths of winter. Other evergreens such as eucalyptus, bay laurel, larch, or juniper can also add decorative charm to a garland.

YOU WILL NEED

Interlocking plastic garland cages (from a florist's)

Floristry foam (or Oasis), Saran wrap, Floristry stub wires

24in (60cm) length of soft cotton cord
or strong silk ribbon

Evergreens: sprays of variegated holly,
blue pine, and viburnum or bay laurel

Dried teasels and poppy seedheads, Pine cones

Mini pumpkins, Gold spray paint

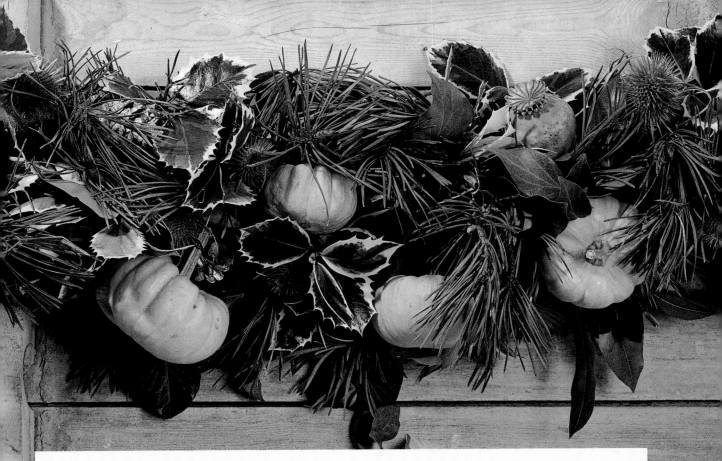

METHOD

❋ Trim the evergreens to equal lengths —
approximately 5in (12cm). Spray some of the teasels
and poppy heads (or the fir cones) gold and leave to
dry thoroughly.

❋ Cut the foam to fit inside the garland cages, then
soak it in water. Cover the foam with Saran wrap
(to help it retain moisture). Insert the foam into the
garland cages.

❋ Cut the length of cotton cord or ribbon in half and
fold each piece into a loop. Attach a loop to each
end of the garland to hang it with.

❋ Bind the evergreen sprigs into small bunches with
stub wires. Starting at one end of the garland, push
the bunches into the cages, ensuring that each
bunch overlaps the next to conceal the wiring and
the cage.

❋ Try to create a balanced and interesting design by
alternating different elements. Continue until the
whole garland is covered.

❋ Finally, wire the poppy seedheads, teasels, pine
cones, and mini pumpkins to the garland with
stub wires.

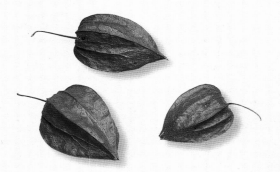

A Kissing Bough

THE TRADITIONAL kissing bough was originally constructed from two bisecting hoops of woven greenery, set with candles and ornamented with items such as colored paper, dried fruit, and sweets. A bunch of mistletoe was suspended from the centre of the hoop, and the bough was then hung from the ceiling of the main living room or hall in the family home. According to legend, mistletoe was considered to be a potent love or fertility charm — hence the custom of kissing under it!

The candles were ceremonially lit for the first time on Christmas Eve and every night thereafter for twelve days. For every kiss given under the bough, one mistletoe berry was removed until all the berries had gone and the kissing had to stop! Today it is still customary to kiss beneath a sprig of mistletoe — yet at one time it was banned by the Christian Church because mistletoe was one of the main sacred plants of the Druids.

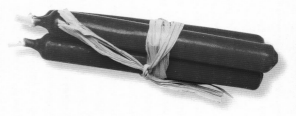

YOU WILL NEED

10in (25cm) twig ring (from florist's)

2¼yd (2m) ¾in (2cm), wide red ribbon

Floristry stub wires

Decorative ribbon tied into bows,
Decorations such as imitation berries and fruits

bundles of tiny red candles tied with raffia colored baubles, 3 red beeswax candles *

Mixed evergreens such as viburnum or bay laurel, blue pine, mistletoe, Dried poppy seedheads, painted red

METHOD

✳ *Twist stub wire round the beeswax candles and push them into the ring.*

✳ *Cut three equal lengths of red ribbon and secure to the ring, leaving an equal space between them, and keeping them away from the candles. Tie the ends together to form a loop to hang the kissing bough.*

✳ *Decorate the ring with the evergreens, weaving them into the twigs. Push the poppy seedheads and the other decorations you have chosen into the ring, using stub wires if necessary.*

✳ *To make your own beeswax candles, use sheets of red beeswax 8in (20cm) square (obtainable from craft shops). Make a sloping cut to trim the top of each sheet from 8in (20cm) at one side to 6in (15cm) at the other. Lay the wick from top to bottom of the sheet at the tallest side. Roll up the beeswax from the tallest side to form a candle.*

✳ *Never leave burning candles unattended.*

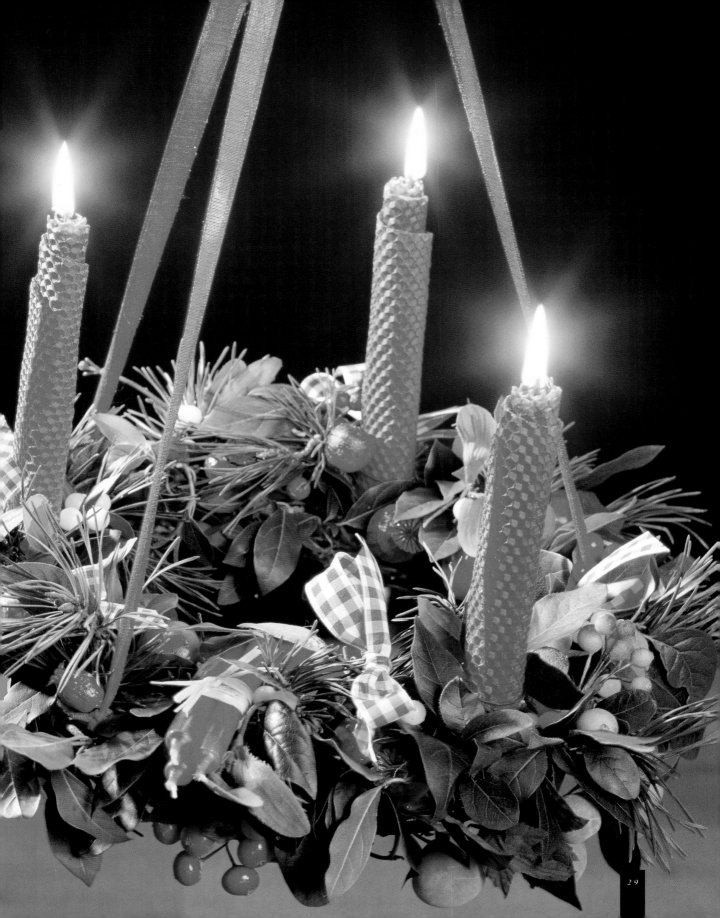

An Aromatic Mobile

IN PARTS OF SCANDINAVIA AND EUROPE, it is customary to make intricate hanging mobiles out of short wheat straws at Christmas time. Dozens of specially prepared straws are threaded together to form stars, pyramids, cones, or other geometric shapes. However, mobiles can be made from all sorts of materials — just use your imagination! They are also a fun and easy project for children. Fir cones, walnuts, shells, feathers, rosehips, cranberries, cardboard shapes, spices, dried fruit, cinnamon sticks, beads, and all sorts of household trinkets can make inspired mobiles. For extra festive appeal, choose lots of aromatic and glittery items.

YOU WILL NEED

Pieces of thin cane (e.g. garden flower sticks)

Floristry wire, Thin gold ribbon,

Gold thread, Transparent thread

Metallic finish gold craft paint

Red and green paint, Glue, Glitter

Large darning needle, A few Brazil nuts

Items for hanging: bay and/or citrus leaves,
small evergreen fronds, small twigs of fir cones,
dried orange and apple rings, dried physalis, thin card,
small Christmas tree decorations

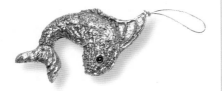

METHOD

❊ Make the main crossbar of the mobile from two equal lengths of cane, crossed over each other and glued. Wire over the top for extra strength. Loop a wire through the center, together with some decorative gold ribbon, from which to hang the mobile.

❊ Cut equal lengths of gold ribbon to suspend from the end of each crossbar. Glue one end of the ribbon to the crossbar. To cover the join, glue a Brazil nut or another decoration over the top. In the same way, fix another gold ribbon to the center of the crossbar. Now collect the items for hanging.

❊ To prepare the orange rings, simply slice a small orange crossways and put the slices on a baking rack to dry out in a very cool oven (110°C/225°F/Gas ¼) for a few hours. Sprinkle a little glitter on them. Apple rings are dried in the same way.

❊ Cut some apple shapes from card, mottle them with red and green paint, then when dry, rub on a little gold paint.

❊ Rub a little gold paint on some of the greenery if you wish.

❊ Attach all the items to the mobile, using gold thread, transparent thread, or wire as necessary. Use the darning needle to thread things on. Some items can be looped directly on to the gold ribbon. Create further "arms" to the mobile by tying on short lengths of cane.

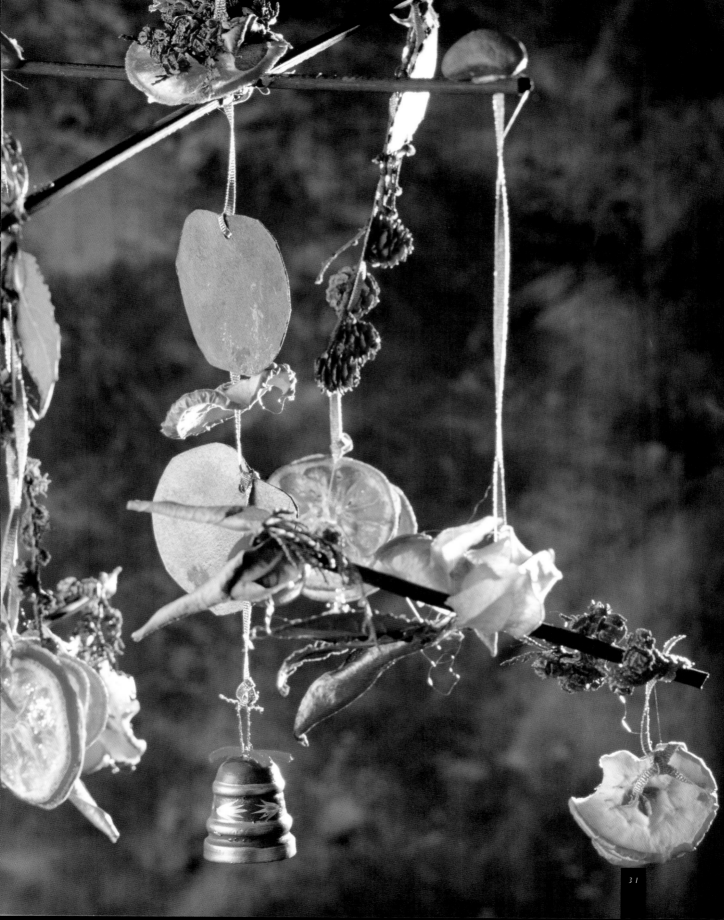

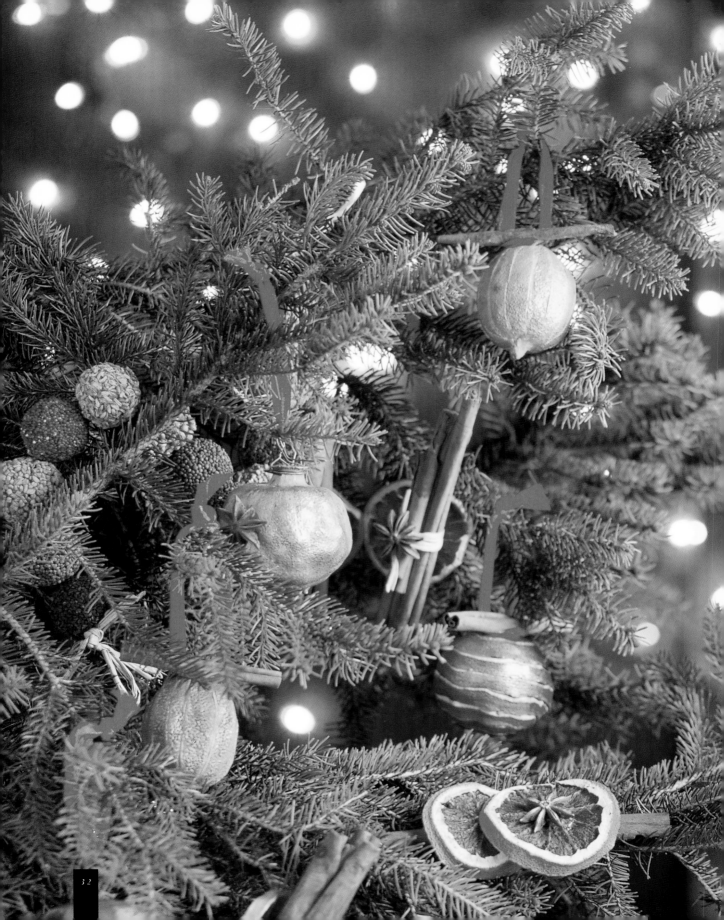

Decorations From Nature

THE DRUIDS BELIEVED that placing evergreen boughs indoors over the winter months provided a safe haven for the tree spirits, who in exchange would ensure that nature was kind to humans. Fruits, spices, and other small edible items were offered as gifts to the tree spirits. Our decorations reflect these ancient beliefs and are very simple to make.

CITRUS GLOBES

YOU WILL NEED Oranges, Lemons
Metallic finish gold craft paint,
Narrow red ribbon, Cinnamon sticks, Glue

✳ *Using a sharp knife, score round the peel of the oranges in a spiral shape. Score the lemon skins lengthways into equal segments.*

✳ *Insert a skewer lengthways through the fruits and balance them above a cookie sheet (which has been lined with silver foil) so the fruit skins are not touching each other or any other surface. Put them in a very cool oven (110°C/225°F/Gas ¼) to dry for several hours until the skins are tough, yet still retain most of their color.*

✳ *Allow the fruits to cool. Rub on a little gold paint.*

✳ *Glue a cinnamon stick to the top of each fruit. Loop some red ribbon under the cinnamon to hang the citrus globe.*

✳ *If you wish, you can sprinkle a few drops of a citrus essential oil on the globes to enhance their fragrance. Seal them in a paper bag, and keep in a warm, dry place for a week before hanging.*

CINNAMON BUNDLES

YOU WILL NEED Cinnamon sticks, Raffia,
Dried star anise pod, Dried orange rings (see pages 30–1)
Metallic finish gold craft paint, Floristry wire, Glue

✳ *Tie a bundle of cinnamon sticks together with raffia. Rub a little gold paint on the star anise slice and glue it to the raffia. Glue a dried orange ring to the opposite side. Loop some wire through the raffia to hang the cinnamon bundle.*

CASSIA BARS

YOU WILL NEED Cassia sticks (from florists),
Dried orange rings (see pages 30–1), Dried star anise pods,
Metallic finish gold craft paint,
Glue, Transparent thread

✳ *Glue two overlapping orange rings to the center of the cassia stick. Rub a little gold paint on a star anise slice and glue it to the upper orange ring. Tie some transparent thread to the cassia bar to hang it with.*

GOLDEN POMEGRANATES

YOU WILL NEED Dried pomegranates, Glue,
Metallic finish gold craft paint
Dried star anise pods, Floristry wire, Narrow red ribbon

✳ *Dry the pomegranates in the manner described on pages 30–1. Rub the fruit with gold paint. Glue a star anise slice to the side of each pomegranate. Dab with a little gold paint. Wind one end of a length of wire around the neck of the fruit; bend the other end into a loop. Thread red ribbon through the loop to hang it with.*

Traditional Tree Decorations

THE GERMANS WERE THE FIRST to display fir trees in their homes at Christmas time, in the sixteenth century. Martin Luther, the leader of the Reformation movement, was reputedly inspired to put the first candles on a Christmas tree after looking at a starry sky while walking through an evergreen forest.

In the middle of the nineteenth century, Prince Albert, the German husband of Queen Victoria, introduced the Christmas tree to England, from where the custom quickly spread to the USA. Early tree decorations – dried fruits, nuts, gingerbread, sweets, and paper roses – were all prepared at home in readiness for dressing the tree on Christmas Eve. Today, although the shops are now full of glittering ready-made decorations, home-made items still have a charm and simplicity which is difficult to match.

CRANBERRY GARLAND AND RINGS

YOU WILL NEED Cranberries or rosehips
Strong thread, Floristry wire

✳ *Using strong thread and a sharp needle, thread the cranberries lengthways into a long chain. Knot the ends securely. Drape over the Christmas tree. To make rings, thread the berries on to wire, shape into a circle and twist the ends together.*

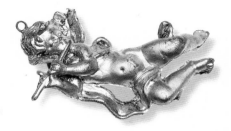

SNOWFLAKES

YOU WILL NEED Paper doilies,
Transparent, Self-adhesive paper, Gold or silver paint
Glitter, Gold or silver thread

✳ *Cut snowflake shapes from the doilies, and paint them gold or silver. Stick them to the self-adhesive paper. Sprinkle with glitter, which will stick to the self-adhesive paper showing through the holes of each doily. Cut round each completed snowflake, and tie to the tree with gold or silver thread.*

DOUGH DECORATIONS

YOU WILL NEED Ready-prepared craft dough
(or make your own from flour and water)
Cookie cutters in Christmas shapes, Paints,
Narrow red and green ribbons

✳ *Roll out the dough, and using the cookie cutters, cut out shapes such as snowmen. Make a small hole to hang with. Dry according to the manufacturer's instructions. Paint each decoration, and hang from the tree with colored ribbon.*

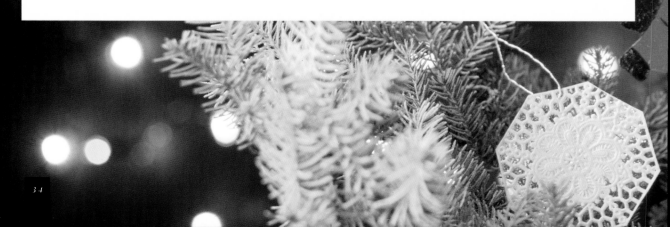

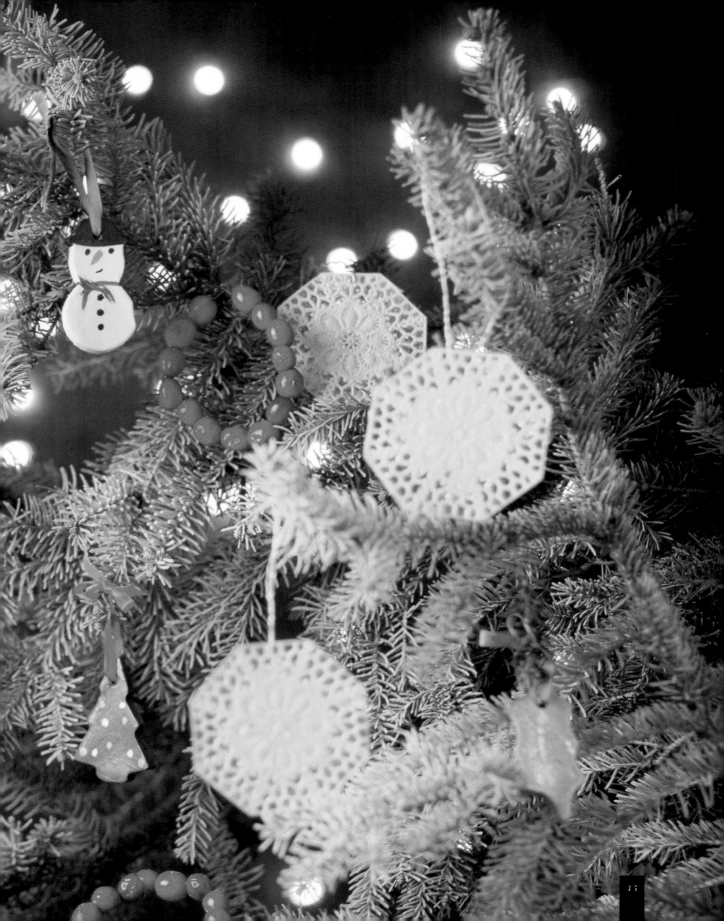

Dried Apple And Spice Ring

MANY OF THE TRADITIONAL Yuletide dishes such as mince pies, spiced biscuits, Christmas cake, and Christmas pudding are baked with dried fruit and spices. At one time, most fresh fruits, herbs, and vegetables were unavailable during the winter months. Dried fruit, which could be stored all the year round, was used instead. These rich, spicy dishes were also warming and sustaining to the body during the coldest period of the year.

The evocative scents of eastern spices such as nutmeg, cinnamon, clove, and ginger have become associated with the atmosphere of the Christmas season. These spices and many others are all readily available in grocery stores. This beautiful dried apple and spice ring will fill the house with an exotic aroma, especially if it is hung in a warm place such as above the kitchen stove.

YOU WILL NEED

8in (20cm) double wire ring (from florist's), or thick gauge florist's wire to make your own

Orange cellophane ribbon, Decorative ribbon

Large red apples, 1¼ cups/½pt (300ml) lemon juice

1¼ cups/½pt (300ml) rosewater

2oz /2 tblsp (60g) salt, 2 tblsp (30ml) citric acid

Dried orange rings, Glue

Cardamom pods, Dried star anise pod, 2 nutmegs

Spicy essential oils, such as cinnamon, anise, clove, nutmeg (optional)

METHOD

✻ Mix the salt, lemon juice and citric acid in a large bowl. Carefully cut the apples crosswise into ¼in (5mm) slices. Soak these in the lemon juice mixture for about five minutes. Toss in rosewater for five minutes. Dry the apples on paper towels than lay them on wire cake racks. Dry them in a very cool oven (110°C/225°F/Gas mark ¼) for six to eight hours until they are a uniform leathery texture.

✻ Take the wire ring, or make your own using the florist's wire, winding and twisting it around to form a circle 12-15in (30-38cm) in diameter. Attach a decorative ribbon securely to this base, to hang it when it is finished.

✻ Bind the ring with the cellophane ribbon, glueing the ends down to secure them. Glue on dried orange rings about ¾in (1.5cm) apart. In the gaps between them, glue the apple rings.

✻ Glue the star anise to the center of one apple ring. Glue five cardamom pods in a star shape in the center of each of the other apple rings. Glue the nutmegs on the opposite side of the ring to the star anise.

✻ Scrunch up some more cellophane ribbon, and glue it to the back of the ring, creating a frilled effect at the inner and outer edges.

✻ To enhance the fragrance of the ring, add 10-12 drops of a spicy-scented essential oil to the ring, and seal in a plastic bag for one or two weeks before displaying it.

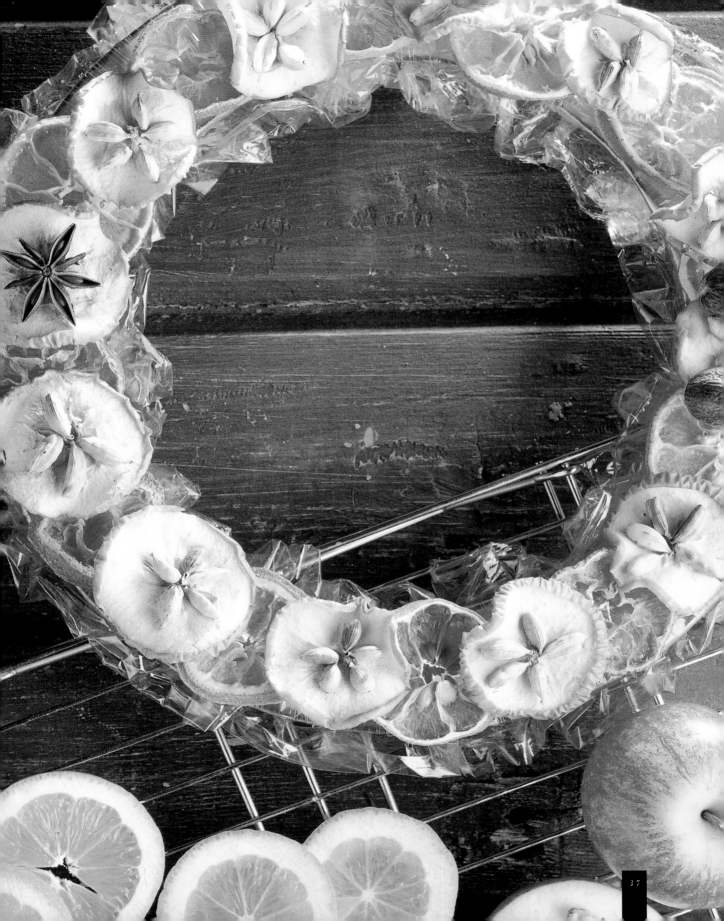

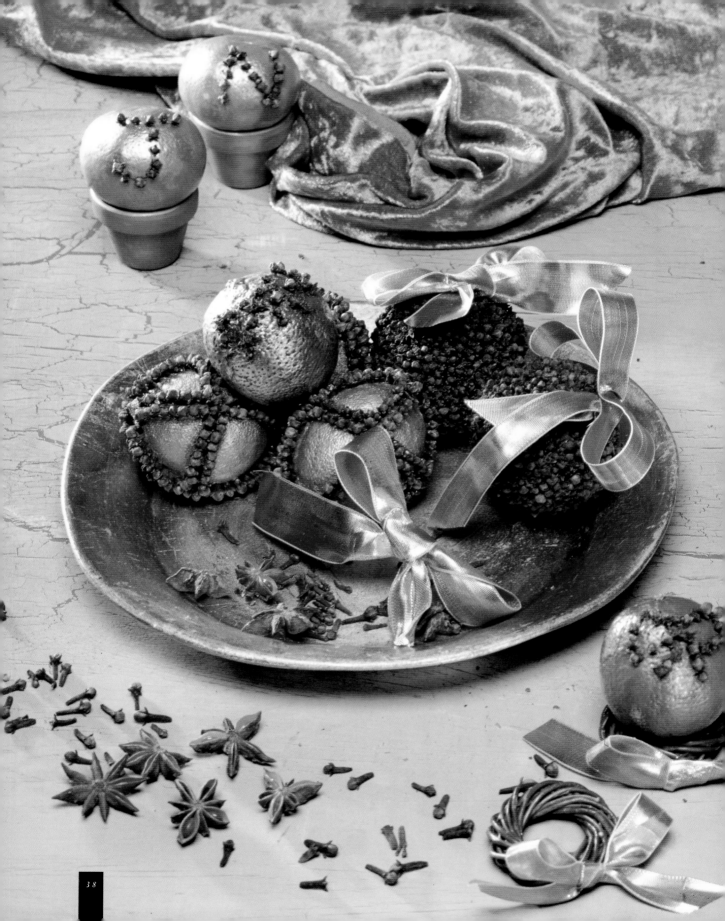

Citrus Pomanders

A POMANDER IS A SOLID BALL of scented materials, originally worn around the neck or at the waist as a type of perfume, or used to ward off infection. Pomanders traditionally contained ambergris, giving rise to the name *pomme ambre* or "amber apple." Later the Arabs introduced to Europe the idea of an orange stuck with cloves or stuffed with medicinal herbs, the latter sometimes soaked in vinegar.

Fruit-based pomanders of this type are highly decorative hung from a ribbon and displayed on the Christmas tree, or grouped together in bowls to form a table centerpiece. They emit a deliciously warming, spicy citrus fragrance.

YOU WILL NEED

Several Seville oranges (and/or tangerines, lemons or limes)

7oz (200g) large whole cloves

Masking or adhesive tape

Clove and orange essential oils

Metallic finish gold craft paint

Length of ¾in (1.5cm) bronze ribbon

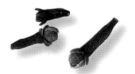

METHOD

✳ *Decide on the design you are going to make with the cloves, and put masking tape on the fruit in the area of the design. Using a skewer or knitting needle, prick holes for the cloves about ¼in (5mm) apart, keeping them evenly spaced. Push whole cloves into the holes one by one, inserting them right up to their heads.*

✳ *You can use your imagination to create any design you wish. We have shown:*
Fruit completely covered with cloves.
Orb design — double rows of cloves stuck lengthways and widthways.
Small bow shapes.
Initials. These make good place indicators for your guests at the festive table.

✳ *Remove the strips of tape, and place the fruit in an airing cupboard or on a radiator for up to a month, turning them occasionally. When they have completely dried out, apply three drops of each essential oil to each fruit, and seal in a bag for one to two weeks.*

✳ *Rub some gold paint over the fruit.*

✳ *Tie the bronze ribbon into decorative bows, and use a pin to secure to the fruit for a finishing touch.*

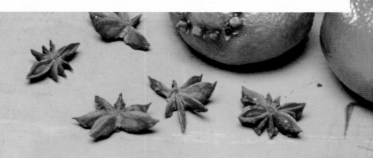

A Burning Perfume

THOUSANDS OF YEARS AGO, incense was used in many cultures as an intrinsic part of sacred rites and rituals, having both a therapeutic and symbolic significance. One well-known incense recipe is found in the Bible, given to Moses (1 part myrrh, 5 parts frankincense and 2½ parts benzoin). The gifts of frankincense and myrrh offered by the Three Kings to the newborn baby Jesus showed their high value as incense materials.

Today, incense still plays a central role in many religious ceremonies, both in the Orient and in the West. During Roman Catholic mass, grains of frankincense are burned to create clouds of fragrant smoke, signifying the communion between the temporal and the divine, the material and immaterial.

Our Christmas burning perfume is also based on frankincense, drawing on this ancient tradition of using fragrance to mark important religious occasions.

YOU WILL NEED

4 parts frankincense essential oil

3 parts cypress essential oil

2 parts orange essential oil

1 part myrrh /clove /cinnamon leaf essential oil

METHOD

✳ *Carefully measure out the essential oils in drops. Seal in a decorative, dark glass bottle and leave to mature for at least two weeks. This mixture can be used as a room fragrance (on a light bulb ring or ceramic burner), or for scenting all manner of items such as paper, pot-pourri, or ribbons.*

✳ *An innovative way of enjoying the burning perfume is to make your own oil burner, using an orange. Take a large fresh orange and cut it in half crosswise. Scoop out the fleshy inside of one half, leaving the central strand of pith intact. Place this in a very cool oven (110°C/225°F/Gas ¼) for six to eight hours, until the peel is completely dry and impenetrable. Now fill the orange with vegetable oil, leaving the top of the white pith just protruding — this will act as a wick. Put several drops of the burning perfume into the oil before lighting the wick. As a room fragrancer, this home-made oil lamp can help create an uplifting, yet soothing effect on Christmas Day!*

✳ *Do not leave burning perfume unattended.*

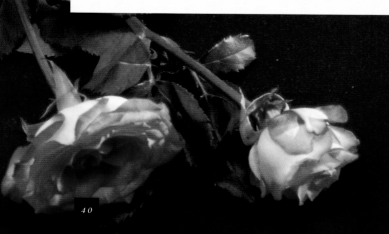

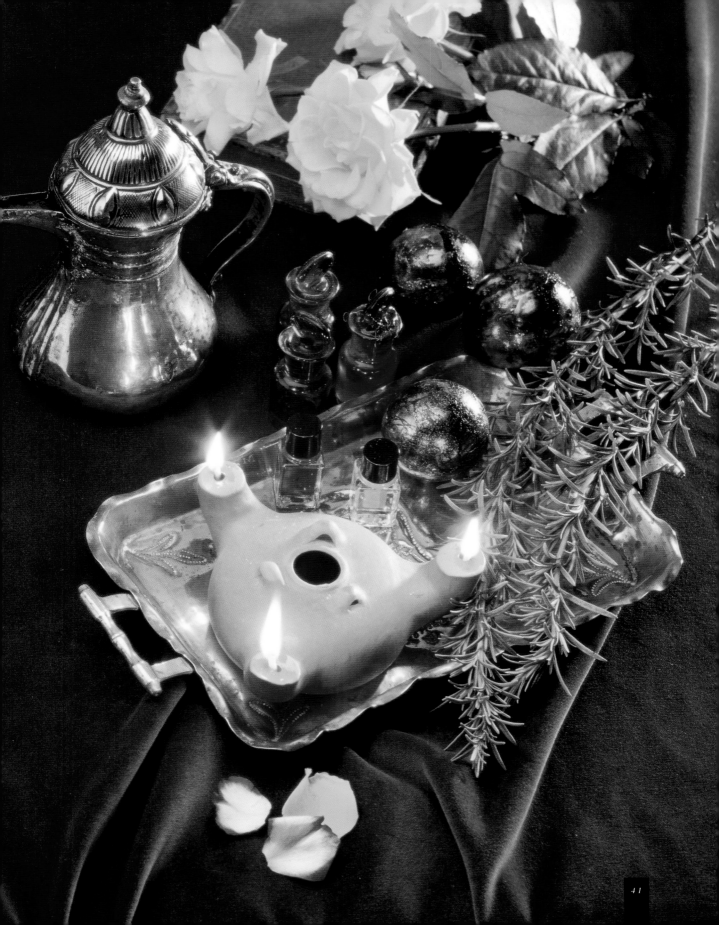

Traditional Christmas Crackers

TOM SMITH, A LONDON PASTRY COOK, is credited with having invented the first crackers in the early 1840s, after a trip to Paris. It was there that he came across fragrant bon-bons wrapped in brightly colored paper with the ends twisted together. His first crackers, called "cosaques," were sweets concealed inside slips of paper printed with different mottoes, wrapped in decorative paper.

The idea was a great success at society parties, so Smith developed the idea still further. Inspired by the crackling of an open fire and by the Chinese custom of setting off fireworks during festivals, he incorporated a "bang" into the cracker when it was pulled. Later on, surprise gifts, jokes, and paper hats were included. One of the most popular Victorian crackers was for spinsters and contained a wedding ring, a bottle of hair dye, and a nightcap!

YOU WILL NEED

For each cracker:

Thin card or ready-made cardboard tube 4½in (11cm) long x 2in (4.5cm) diameter

Colored tissue paper, Colored cellophane

Writing paper, Glue, Narrow glittery ribbon

Decorations: bay leaves, stick-on jewels, dried lavender, and marjoram flowers

Peppermints

For the peppermints:

1 egg white, A few drops of peppermint essence

3 cups/12oz (300g) sieved icing sugar (confectioner's sugar)

METHOD

✶ Cut the thin card into a rectangle 4⅓in (11cm) x 6in (15cm). Put a few peppermints on it and roll it up into a tube, then secure it with a rubber band, Scotch tape or glue.

✶ Cut a small slip of writing paper and write on a personal message, joke, motto or short quotation. Push the message into the tube.

✶ Now cut the tissue paper into a 11⅓in (29cm) x 6½in (16.5cm) strip. Cut the cellophane to the same size, then snip the long sides into a deep zigzag shape.

✶ Place the tissue paper on to the cellophane. With the cellophane on the outside, wrap both round the cardboard tube and roll up. Secure the end with a piece of double sided tape in the center.

✶ Scrunch the tissue paper and cellophane together at the ends of the tube, and tie with narrow glittery ribbon.

✶ Decorate the body of the cracker by sticking on the decorations. Open the crackers at the end of the meal to enjoy the peppermints.

TO MAKE THE PEPPERMINTS

✶ Whisk the egg white until frothy, then gradually beat in the sugar. Add peppermint essence to taste, before the mixture gets too stiff. Knead it until it is a smooth consistency. Dust a board with a little of the sugar and turn the mixture on to it. Roll out the paste and use a small cutter to make rounds (or other shapes). Dry on a rack for about twelve hours. Makes three dozen.

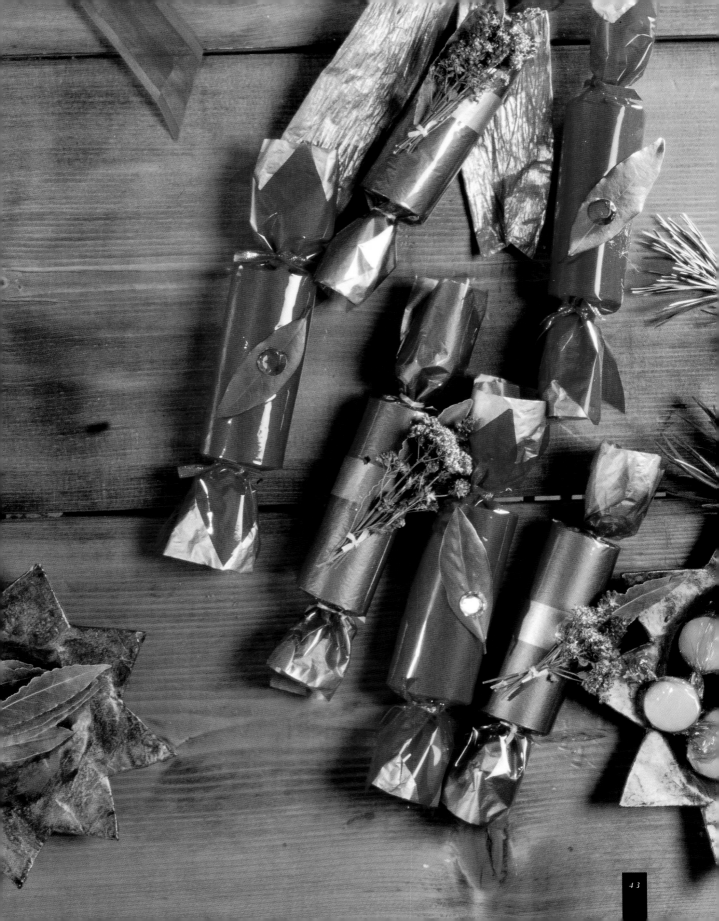

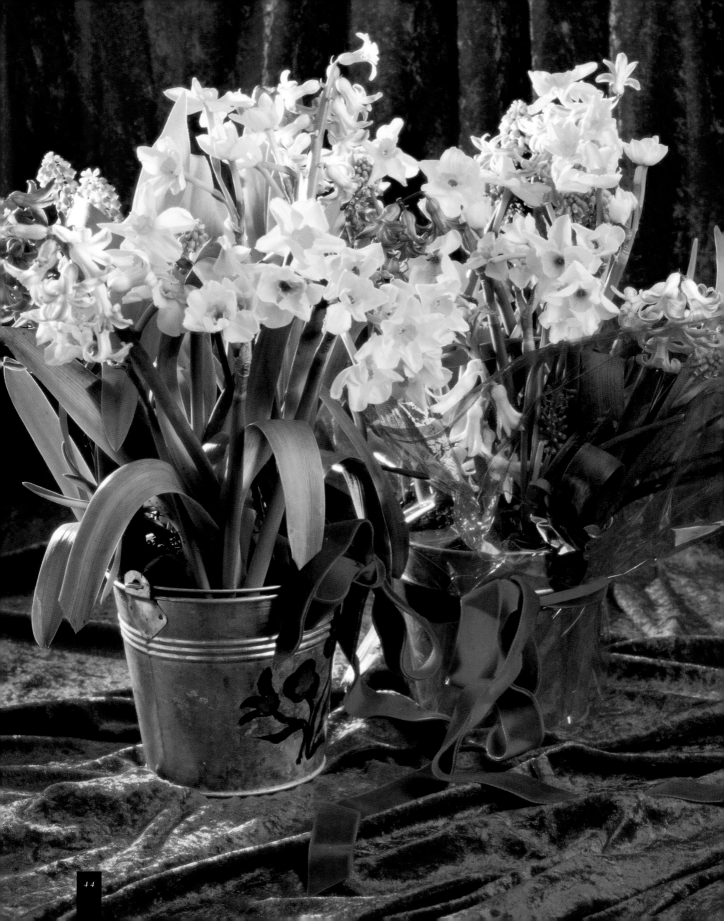

Fresh Scented Flowers

IT IS CONSIDERED UNLUCKY to leave Christmas decorations in place beyond January 6th. Flowers, however, effortlessly blur the boundary between a Christmas display and one which is appropriate for the New Year. Flowers are the archetypal harbingers of spring, and in the mythology of all civilizations alike, the emergence of the first buds after the hardship of winter is a universal symbol of renewal.

Flowers which bloom in the winter take on a special significance when most other plants are dormant. Many types of bulb can be forced to flower indoors: the best scented varieties for forcing include hyacinths, paperwhite narcissi, and dwarf irises. Other spring-flowering bulbs normally grown outside, such as snowdrops, crocuses, and scillas, can be encouraged to flower earlier by bringing them indoors into the warmth.

YOU WILL NEED

Bulbs, such as blue and pink hyacinths, red tulips, muscari, narcissi

Two aluminum buckets

Two flowerpots to fit the buckets

Bulb fibre, Ceramic paints

Purple cellophane

Purple velvet ribbon 1in (2.5cm) wide

METHOD

✱ *For flowers at Christmas, start this project in the fall. Check how long the bulbs you have chosen for forcing will need to come into flower (around two months).*

✱ *Cover the drainage hole and the bottom of the flowerpots with a layer of broken crocks or pebbles. Fill the pots with bulb fiber, then plant a selection of bulbs in each pot.*

✱ *Put the pots in a cool, dark place for about five weeks, then bring them out into a light, warmish 10°C (50°F) room — if it is too hot or too dark the plants will become leggy.*

✱ *Put the flowerpots into the aluminum buckets. We painted one with ceramic paints in a floral design; the other was wrapped in purple cellophane, cinched with a purple velvet ribbon. Use thin canes and ribbons to support the flower heads if they become too tall or heavy.*

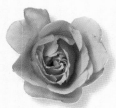
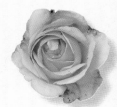

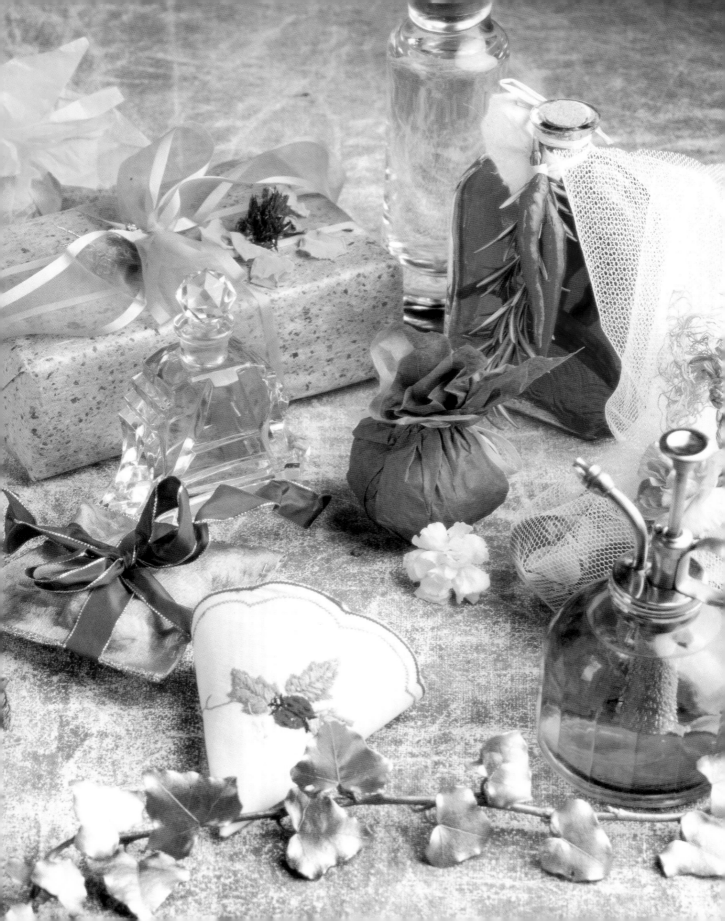

PART TWO

Fragrant Gifts

A LARGE PART OF THE MAGIC AND JOY of Christmas is in the anticipation! This is especially true where children are concerned. Decorating the house with evergreens and brightly colored lights, making mince pies, dressing the Christmas tree, wrapping gifts and, of course, counting the days until they can unwrap their own presents, are undoubtedly high points in any child's year.

Generosity towards others is also an intrinsic part of the Christmas spirit. Boxing Day is said to derive its name from the alms boxes which were placed in churches over the festive period, the contents of which were distributed among the poor on the day after Christmas.

The celebration of Christmas and the exchange of gifts need not be an expensive affair. Plants gathered from the garden or countryside, scraps of fabric, old Christmas cards, empty jars or bottles and other types of household junk can all be transformed, with a little bit of imagination, into unique and personalized gifts. It may require more time and planning than buying presents from a shop, but the greatest pleasure can be gained by making all kinds of original presents at home. For example, jars of home-made preserved fruits, or fragrant oils and vinegars, are always more welcome than shop-bought commercial varieties.

LEFT: There are lots of ways of capturing a natural scent.

RIGHT: A handmade gift says a great deal about a friendship.

The following pages contain a wealth of creative ideas, some innovative, and others with a traditional theme. There is something for everyone. Children will enjoy making items such as pot-pourri (using petals gathered from the garden), and scented Christmas cards. Above all, it is the fun and satisfaction of creating things with your own hands that can help to recreate the true spirit of Christmas, both within the family and between friends.

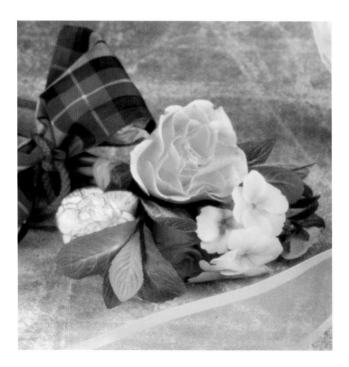

"I will keep Christmas in the cold hedgerow, With shining holly and winter snow. Stars will be candles of sweet silver fire, swinging at midnight over tree and spire."

Scented Christmas Cards

THE SHOPS ARE FULL of a vast range of colorful cards at Christmas, yet there is nothing like receiving a personalized card which has been hand-made or printed at home. Most children enjoy making cards in the weeks preceding Christmas, using simple potato blocks or ready-made stamps (available from craft shops). Exciting effects can also be achieved by laying hand-cut paper stencils on to a piece of card, then spraying with gold or silver spray paint. Sequins, glitter glue, pieces of metallic foil or shiny stickers can be added to give the designs a festive feel. Interesting leaves, or flat seed pods sprayed gold, can also be stuck on.

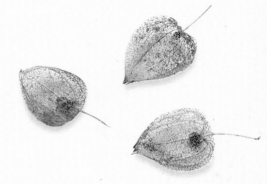

YOU WILL NEED

Various types of card

Decorative items (see individual suggestions)

Cotton pad, Essential oil

Airtight container

METHOD

✳ *Make your Christmas cards — follow our suggestions, or improvise.*

✳ *Impregnate the cotton pad with a few drops of essential oil, and put it into the container, together with the Christmas cards. Seal, and leave for seven to ten days for the cards to absorb the perfume.*

✳ *Starry sky card. Use green corrugated card, stamped with gold star shapes (use a potato or ready-made stamp). Glue decorative ribbon to the spine, folding the ends underneath to neaten.*

✳ *Yellow parcel card. Fold a piece of yellow corrugated card into an envelope shape. Place two dried orange rings in the envelope. Tie the parcel together with cheerful checked red ribbon.*

✳ *Apple spice card. Use pink card, cut with a zigzag edge. Brush patches with glue and sprinkle glitter on. Glue a dried apple ring to the center. Punch two holes in each side edge of the card, and knot together with cord.*

✳ *Star of Bethlehem card. Fold a piece of cream corrugated card. Stamp the front at the lower center with a gold star. Tie a bow from pink sheer ribbon and glue on. Brush a little gold paint or glitter on to the bow.*

✳ *Evergreen bouquet card. Take a piece of buff-colored corrugated card and fold. Cut a window in the front, and glue a piece of green card to it. Tie a thin red ribbon round a sprig of evergreen and mini fir cones. Glue to the green window. Glue a gold ribbon bow at the side of the card.*

✳ *Ribbon rose card. Fold a piece of cream corrugated card. To the front, glue a dried rose, bay leaves painted gold, and a checked ribbon bow. Glue a strip of checked ribbon to the back as a hanger.*

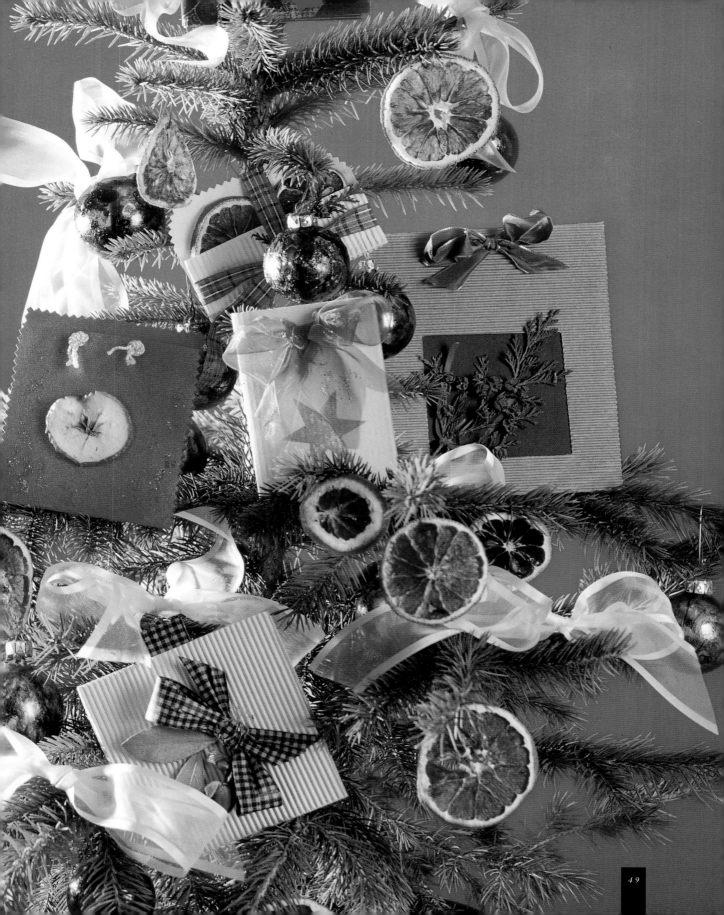

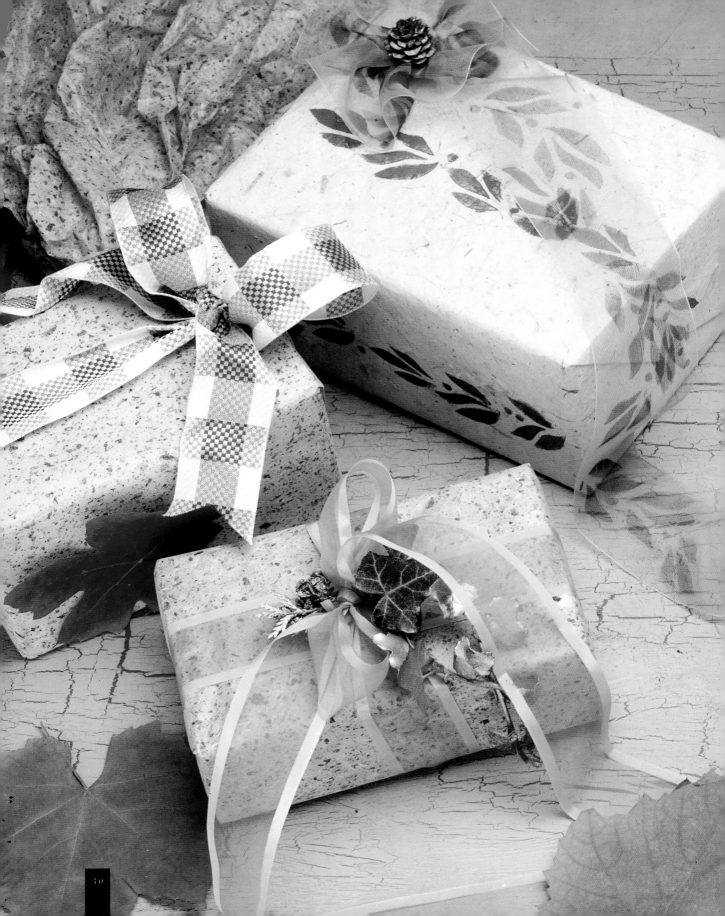

Perfumed Wrappings

THE WRAPPING OF PRESENTS is synonymous with the rituals of Christmas. It's a tradition which relies on elements of anticipation, mystery and secrecy for its age-old popularity. Paper, ribbons, and tags can also be scented to enhance their appeal.

It is easy to make your own wrapping paper at home using a variety of different techniques. Try printing paper with simple potato block cuts. Another effective decoration is to lay leaves on the paper, then spray over them with gold spray paint, to leave subtle outlines. A similar effect can be achieved by laying a paper doily on brightly colored tissue paper, before spraying it with gold or silver paint.

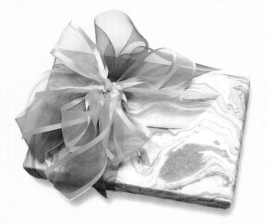

ABOVE: Parcel wrapped in marbled paper, tied with mauve sheer ribbon (2½in/6cm wide). Decorated with three bows – one of mauve sheer ribbon and two of cream sheer ribbon.

METHOD

✳ Paper, ribbons and leaves can be scented before use with essential oils. Shake a few drops of the essential oil on to a piece of cloth. Put the cloth, paper and other items together in a sealed container for at least one week prior to using them.

✳ Bay leaf wrapping (handmade paper stencilled with bay leaf design). Stencil or paint on the bay leaves in a "ribbon" across the paper. Stencil the same design on to the sheer ribbon. Gather and sew a piece of the ribbon to make a rosette, then glue the fir cone in the center. Wrap the parcel, and decorate with the ribbon and rosette.

✳ Maple leaf wrapping (beige and gold paper, checked ribbon). Wrap the parcel. Tie the ribbon into a bow, and glue on. Glue on the pressed maple leaf to decorate.

✳ Ivy leaf wrapping (beige and gold paper, sheer ribbon). Wrap the parcel. Tie the sheer ribbon round the parcel in the traditional cross shape. Glue the ivy and cypress sprays to the center of the cross. Tie a separate bow from the sheer ribbon and glue over the ivy and cypress.

YOU WILL NEED

Essential oil, such as pine, cypress, cinnamon, or orange

Bay leaf wrapping: handmade paper, stencil, green paint, 2½in (6cm) wide sheer ribbon, tiny fir cone (sprayed gold), glue

Maple leaf wrapping: beige and gold speckled paper, 1½in (4cm) wide brown and cream checked ribbon, pressed maple leaf, glue

Ivy leaf wrapping: beige and gold speckled paper, 1½in (4cm) wide sheer ribbon, small stems of ivy and cypress (sprayed gold), glue

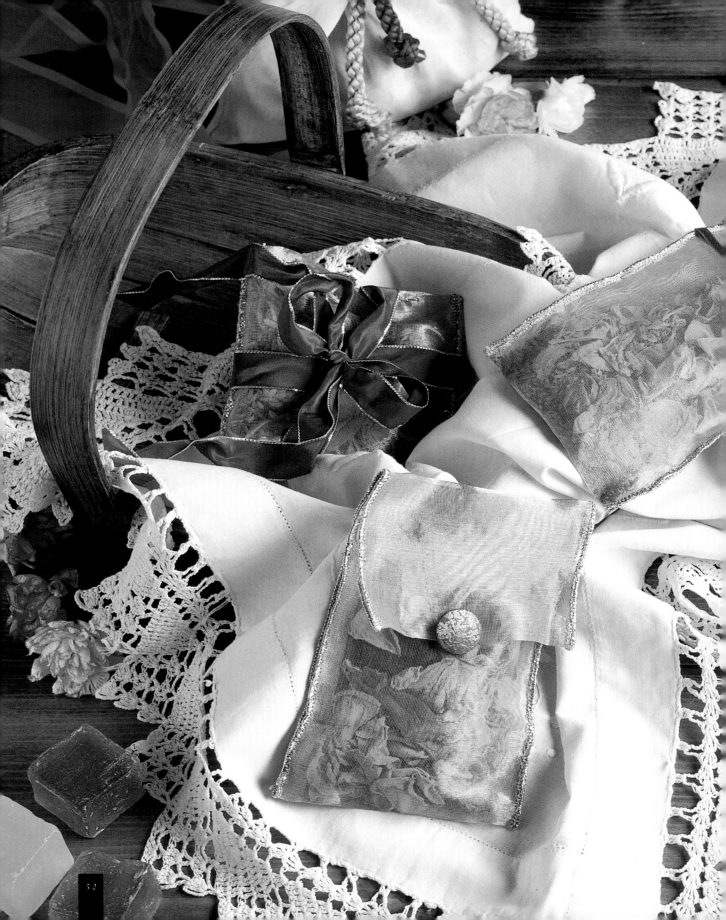

Tussie Mussies

A TUSSIE MUSSIE IS a small scented bouquet, which (like the pomander) was originally used hundreds of years ago to help combat unpleasant odors when soap and water were luxuries. In medieval times, fragrant herbs such as rosemary, sage, rue, wormwood, and lavender were thought to prevent the spread of contagious disease, and it was common to carry a posy of herbs strung from the belt to ward off infection. In the sixteenth century, the tussie mussie developed as a more romantic notion — the gift of a fragrant posy was used as a means of exchanging messages between lovers, secretly conveyed in the universally understood "language of flowers." Each bloom or sprig carried its own message: rosemary, for example, represented faithfulness or remembrance, roses declared love, lavender stated silence, marjoram wished fruitfulness, and marigolds beamed happiness.

YOU WILL NEED
FOR FRESH TUSSIE MUSSIES

Freesias, Blue hyacinths, Roses,

Pinks, Primulas, Common primroses,

Mint, Fennel, Marjoram,

Rosemary, Chives, Raffia,

METHOD

✳ *Make small posies from a selection of flowers and herbs. Bind the stems together with raffia.*

✳ *Tussie mussies can also be made from a selection of dried flowers and herbs. Bind the stems together with floristry wire. Push each posy through the center of a doily and secure with a decorative ribbon. Drip a few drops of an essential oil into the interior of the posy. Place the posy in a sealed brown paper bag, away from light and heat, for at least two weeks.*

By Victorian times, the arrangement had become quite formal, consisting of concentric rings of leaves, sprigs of herbs, and scented flowers encircling a central bud, usually a rose. Slowly, as the symbolism of the tussie mussie faded, it was offered as a gift on all sorts of occasions including weddings, funerals, and at Easter and Christmas.

A posy gathered fresh from the garden makes a charming present, but in winter you may need to resort to a florist's shop. Tussie mussies may also be made from dried flowers and herbs to create a more enduring gift.

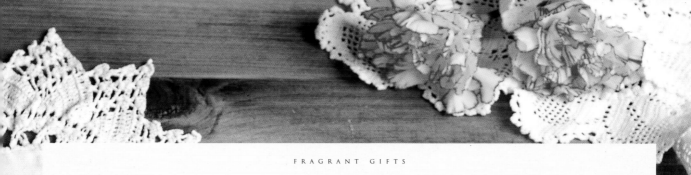

Lavender Bags

DRIED LAVENDER IS one of the most versatile aromatic materials and has been used for centuries to protect clothes and linen from moths, at the same time infusing the material with a delicate, soothing fragrance. Lavender bags can be slipped into a clothes drawer, hung in the wardrobe or placed in the linen cupboard. In Victorian times, a heart-shaped lavender sachet, made from net and tied with velvet ribbon, was the traditional gift of a maiden aunt to her young nieces! Lavender bags are a delightful Christmas gift when made from festive ribbons.

In summer, pick lavender (with a good length of stem) just before it comes into full bloom, on a warm day. Hang small bunches to dry in a dark, ventilated place – an old cupboard is ideal – or lay out on trays lined with newspaper and slide under a bed or chest of drawers.

YOU WILL NEED

4oz (100g) dried lavender flowers
(or use rosemary or ground cloves)

1oz (25g) orris root powder

5 drops lavender essential oil
(or use cedarwood, rosemary, or clove)

Gold sheer wire-edged ribbon, 3in (8cm) wide

Gold-edged blue ribbon, 1in (2cm) wide

Narrow red ribbon, Gold button

METHOD

✳ *Mix the dried flowers with the orris root powder and add the essential oil. Seal in an airtight container and allow the mixture to mature for at least one week.*

✳ *Place a handful of the scented mixture in each lavender bag, made as follows.*

✳ **Bag 1**. *Cut a 10in (25cm) length of the gold sheer ribbon. Turn the ends in and stitch. Stitch three strips of red ribbon to one end of the gold ribbon, turning under the ends. Fold the gold ribbon in two and stitch up the sides to form the bag. Put the dried flowers inside, and catch-stitch the ends of the bag together.*

✳ **Bag 2**. *Cut a 13in (32cm) length of gold sheer ribbon. Neaten the ends as for bag 1. Fold 5½in (14cm) of the ribbon over on itself, and stitch the sides together. Put the lavender into the pocket. Fold over the remaining 2in (4cm) to make the pocket flap. Sew the gold button to the pocket to secure the flap.*

✳ **Bag 3**. *Cut a 8in (20cm) length of gold sheer ribbon. Turn in the ends, then fold in half and stitch up the sides. Fill with lavender. Catch-stitch the ends of the bag together. Tie the lavender bag like a parcel with the gold-edged blue ribbon.*

Scented Christmas Cards

THE SHOPS ARE FULL of a vast range of colorful cards at Christmas, yet there is nothing like receiving a personalized card which has been hand-made or printed at home. Most children enjoy making cards in the weeks preceding Christmas, using simple potato blocks or ready-made stamps (available from craft shops). Exciting effects can also be achieved by laying hand-cut paper stencils on to a piece of card, then spraying with gold or silver spray paint. Sequins, glitter glue, pieces of metallic foil or shiny stickers can be added to give the designs a festive feel. Interesting leaves, or flat seed pods sprayed gold, can also be stuck on.

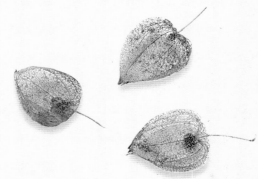

YOU WILL NEED

Various types of card

Decorative items (see individual suggestions)

Cotton pad, Essential oil

Airtight container

METHOD

✻ *Make your Christmas cards — follow our suggestions, or improvise.*

✻ *Impregnate the cotton pad with a few drops of essential oil, and put it into the container, together with the Christmas cards. Seal, and leave for seven to ten days for the cards to absorb the perfume.*

✻ *Starry sky card. Use green corrugated card, stamped with gold star shapes (use a potato or ready-made stamp). Glue decorative ribbon to the spine, folding the ends underneath to neaten.*

✻ *Yellow parcel card. Fold a piece of yellow corrugated card into an envelope shape. Place two dried orange rings in the envelope. Tie the parcel together with cheerful checked red ribbon.*

✻ *Apple spice card. Use pink card, cut with a zigzag edge. Brush patches with glue and sprinkle glitter on. Glue a dried apple ring to the center. Punch two holes in each side edge of the card, and knot together with cord.*

✻ *Star of Bethlehem card. Fold a piece of cream corrugated card. Stamp the front at the lower center with a gold star. Tie a bow from pink sheer ribbon and glue on. Brush a little gold paint or glitter on to the bow.*

✻ *Evergreen bouquet card. Take a piece of buff-colored corrugated card and fold. Cut a window in the front, and glue a piece of green card to it. Tie a thin red ribbon round a sprig of evergreen and mini fir cones. Glue to the green window. Glue a gold ribbon bow at the side of the card.*

✻ *Ribbon rose card. Fold a piece of cream corrugated card. To the front, glue a dried rose, bay leaves painted gold, and a checked ribbon bow. Glue a strip of checked ribbon to the back as a hanger.*

PART TWO

Fragrant Gifts

A LARGE PART OF THE MAGIC AND JOY *of Christmas is in the anticipation! This is especially true where children are concerned. Decorating the house with evergreens and brightly colored lights, making mince pies, dressing the Christmas tree, wrapping gifts and, of course, counting the days until they can unwrap their own presents, are undoubtedly high points in any child's year.*

Generosity towards others is also an intrinsic part of the Christmas spirit. Boxing Day is said to derive its name from the alms boxes which were placed in churches over the festive period, the contents of which were distributed among the poor on the day after Christmas.

The celebration of Christmas and the exchange of gifts need not be an expensive affair. Plants gathered from the garden or countryside, scraps of fabric, old Christmas cards, empty jars or bottles and other types of household junk can all be transformed, with a little bit of imagination, into unique and personalized gifts. It may require more time and planning than buying presents from a shop, but the greatest pleasure can be gained by making all kinds of original presents at home. For example, jars of home-made preserved fruits, or fragrant oils and vinegars, are always more welcome than shop-bought commercial varieties.

LEFT: There are lots of ways of capturing a natural scent.

RIGHT: A handmade gift says a great deal about a friendship.

The following pages contain a wealth of creative ideas, some innovative, and others with a traditional theme. There is something for everyone. Children will enjoy making items such as pot-pourri (using petals gathered from the garden), and scented Christmas cards. Above all, it is the fun and satisfaction of creating things with your own hands that can help to recreate the true spirit of Christmas, both within the family and between friends.

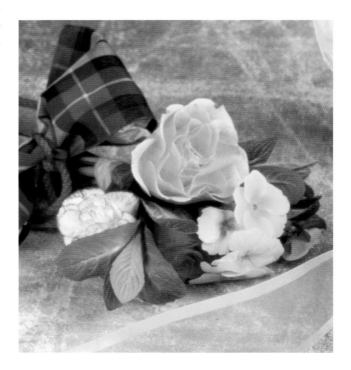

"I will keep Christmas in the cold hedgerow, With shining holly and winter snow. Stars will be candles of sweet silver fire, swinging at midnight over tree and spire."

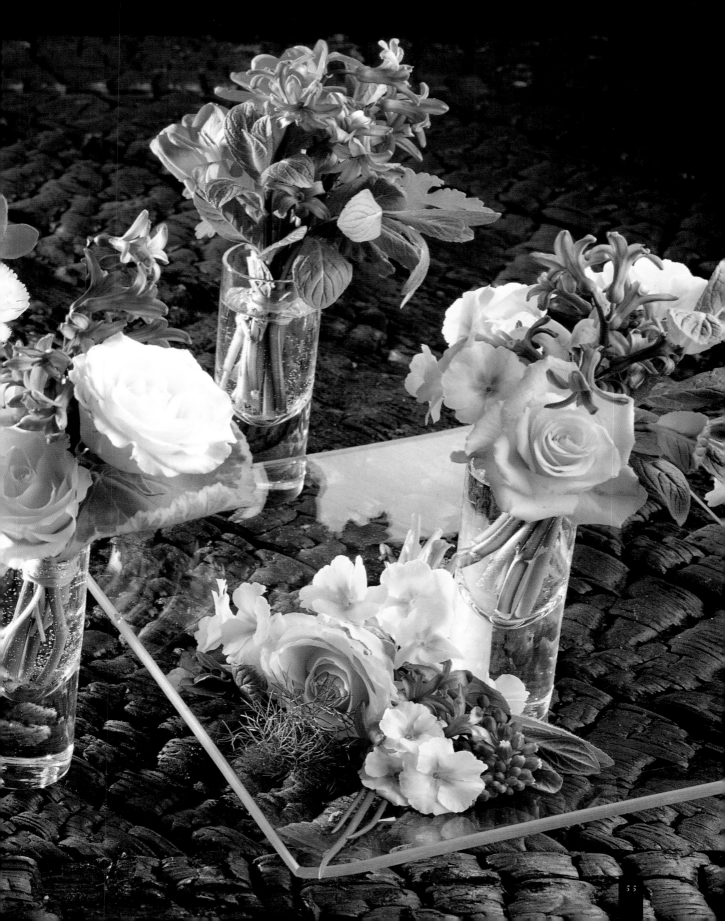

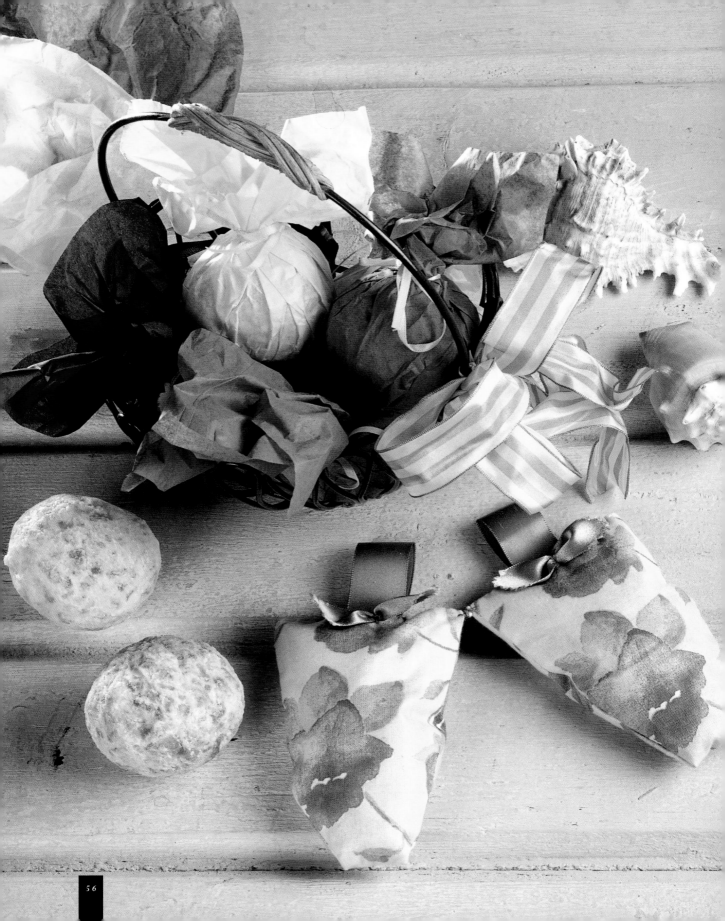

Perfumed Wash Balls

PLANTS HAVE BEEN USED to perfume toilet materials for thousands of years. Lavender has been appreciated for its clean, fresh fragrance since Roman times, while soapwort provided an early form of soap. In the East, rosewater was used to bathe the hands and feet of visitors after a long journey, often presented in ornate vases. In medieval Europe, on major feast days such as Christmas, it was customary to place great bowls of rosewater or other fragrant herbs on the dining table where the guests could wash their hands after eating.

Later, scented wash balls made from Castile soap blended with rosewater and other herbs such as

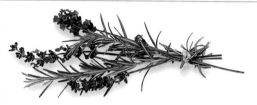

YOU WILL NEED

1 cup/4oz (100g) unscented toilet soap
(or assorted soap ends)

⅔ cup/ 1/4pt (150ml) rosewater

5 drops lavender oil, 5 drops petitgrain oil

Food coloring (optional), Tissue paper

Satin ribbon, ¼in (3mm) wide

METHOD

✳ *Grate the soap into a mixing bowl using a fine grater (such as a cheese grater), then add the rosewater.*

✳ *Heat the mixture over a gentle heat in a bain-marie, until it coalesces into a thick paste. Take it off the heat, and with a pestle and mortar (or blender) mix in the essential oils and food coloring.*

✳ *Allow the mixture to begin to set and dry out a bit, then take a small handful of paste and mold it into a neat ball. Repeat until the mixture is used up. Before the wash balls become completely hard, polish them to a smooth finish by wetting your hands with a little rosewater, and rubbing the balls between them.*

✳ *Wrap each completed wash ball in two 8in (20cm) squares of tissue paper, and tie it with ribbon.*

lavender, cypress or rosemary were prepared in the still room of wealthy houses, along with other aromatic elixirs. Our modern version of these old-fashioned wash balls makes a delightful gift, carefully wrapped in tissue paper. They look lovely piled high in glass jars and displayed in the bathroom.

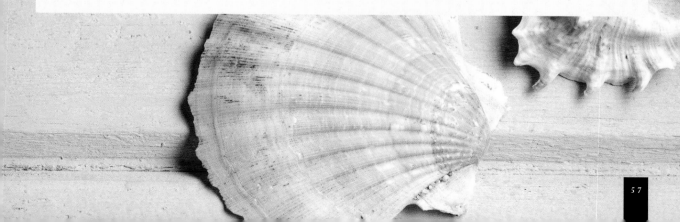

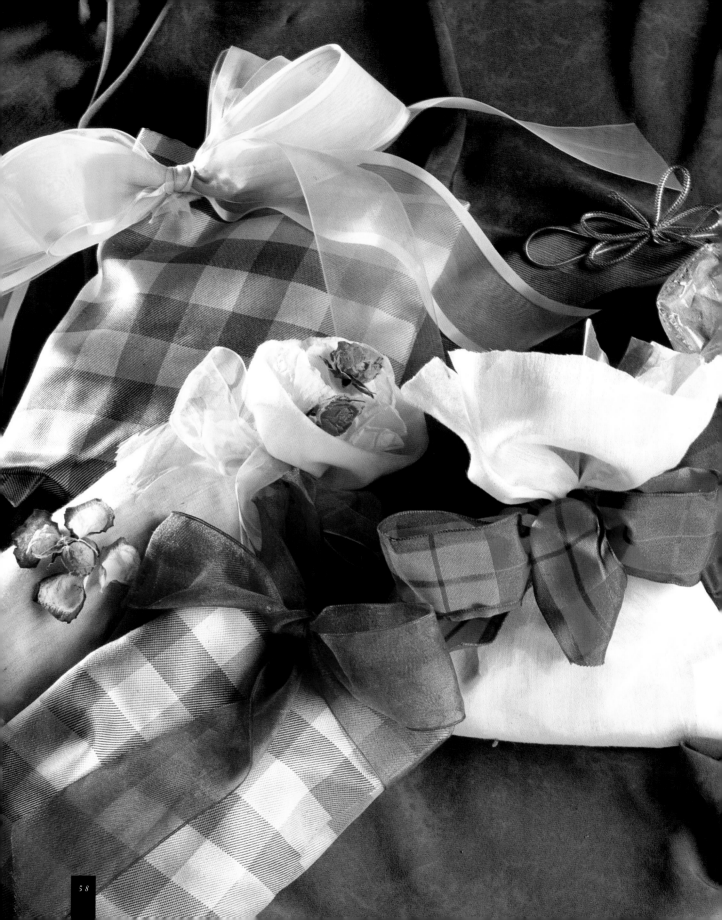

Herb Pillows

AFTER THE HECTIC social rounds of Christmas are over, a fragrant herb pillow will help ensure a restful night's sleep. Herb pillows developed from the practice of stuffing mattresses with scented plants, and from the tradition of using "strewing herbs" such as woodruff and chamomile to cover bare floors with a scented herbal carpet. The Roman emperor, Nero, is said to have slept on a mattress stuffed with fragrant grasses and dried rose petals, while Charles VI of France preferred a lavender-scented bed and pillows.

YOU WILL NEED

1 cup/½oz (12g) dried lavender

1 cup/½oz (12g) dried lemon verbena

1 cup/½oz (12g) dried hops

1 cup/½oz (12g) dried rose petals

1 lightly crushed cinnamon stick

1 tblsp dried cloves

5-10 drops of lavender essential oil

5-10 drops of bergamot essential oil

PLUS, FOR EACH PILLOW:

2 pieces of quilting wadding about 8in (20cm) square

2 pieces of plain cotton about 8in (20cm) square

2 pieces of fabric for the casing (silk, cotton, or tapestry) about 8in (20cm) square

Ribbons, lace or tassels etc. for decoration

METHOD

✳ *Mix the dried herbs, spices and oils together and leave to cure for one to two weeks in a dark, sealed container.*

✳ *Place a piece of wadding on each piece of plain cotton, and sew round all the sides. With the cotton sides together, sew round three sides. Turn the right way out. Stuff the aromatic herb mixture into the sachet through the remaining open side. Finish the fourth side neatly.*

✳ *Now make the outer casing of the pillow in the same manner, placing the right sides of the fabric together, sewing round three sides, and turning the right way out. Leave the fourth side open. Turn the edges of the open side in to neaten. Finish with several ribbons used as ties, or use poppers. Decorate the pillow with lace, tassels or ribbons. Slip the sachet inside.*

Little herb pillows look good piled on sofas or beds, mixed with ordinary pillows. Our recipe for a sleep-inducing pillow has a floral, slightly spicy, festive bouquet. Other suitable dried herbs include mint, lemon balm, chamomile, woodruff and marjoram. For larger sized pillows, dried hops are useful for adding bulk – make sure at least half the contents is herb, though, to keep the scent going.

Sweet Bags

"Take 1lb each of orris roots, sweet calamus, cypress roots, dried lemon peel, dried orange peel and dried roses. Make all these into a gross powder. Take coriander seeds 4oz, nutmegs 1½oz, cloves 1oz; mix them all into a fine powder and then mix with the other. Add musk and ambergris.
Then take four large handfuls of lavender flowers dried and rubbed, a handful each of sweet marjoram, orange leaves and walnut leaves, all dried and rubbed. Mix all together with some bits of cotton perfumed with essences and put it up into silk bags."

THE COMPLEAT HOUSEWIFE, Williamsburg 1742.

SACHETS OF POWDERED AROMATICS, or sweet bags, have been used for centuries to perfume all kind of household items such as gloves, linen and scarves. Indian shawls, for example, were traditionally scented with patchouli oil which not only protected against moths, but also gave a long-lasting fragrance reminiscent of the East. Writing paper, handkerchiefs and underwear can all be imbued with perfume by enclosing them in a sealed container with a mixture of oils and powdered herbs for at least one week. Our sweet bag is based on an eighteenth-century recipe.

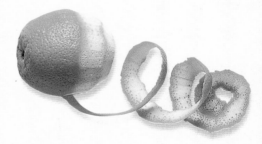

YOU WILL NEED

4 cups/1lb (450g) orris root powder

Handful each of dried lavender, dried marjoram, dried lemon peel, dried orange peel, and dried rose petals

5 cotton pads

30 drops essential oils
(10 each of cypress, clove and nutmeg)

5 purchased circular place mats or dressing table mats 8in (20cm) diameter

Ribbon, 3in (7.5cm) wide

METHOD

❋ Crush the dried herbs to a rough-textured powder, using a pestle and mortar. Add the orris root.

❋ Put two drops of each of the essential oils on to each cotton pad. Place these, together with the crushed herbs, into a tin or sealed jar to cure for one week.

❋ Divide the herb mixture into five equal parts, including a cotton pad with each portion.

❋ Make the sweet bags. Fold each mat in half, then wrap into a cone shape. Sew the edges of the outer layer to secure. Fill the cone with herb mixture. Draw together the inner layers of the cone to enclose the mixture, and sew together. (Alternative bags are made from the ribbon — folded into an envelope, stitched and stuffed with herb mixture.)

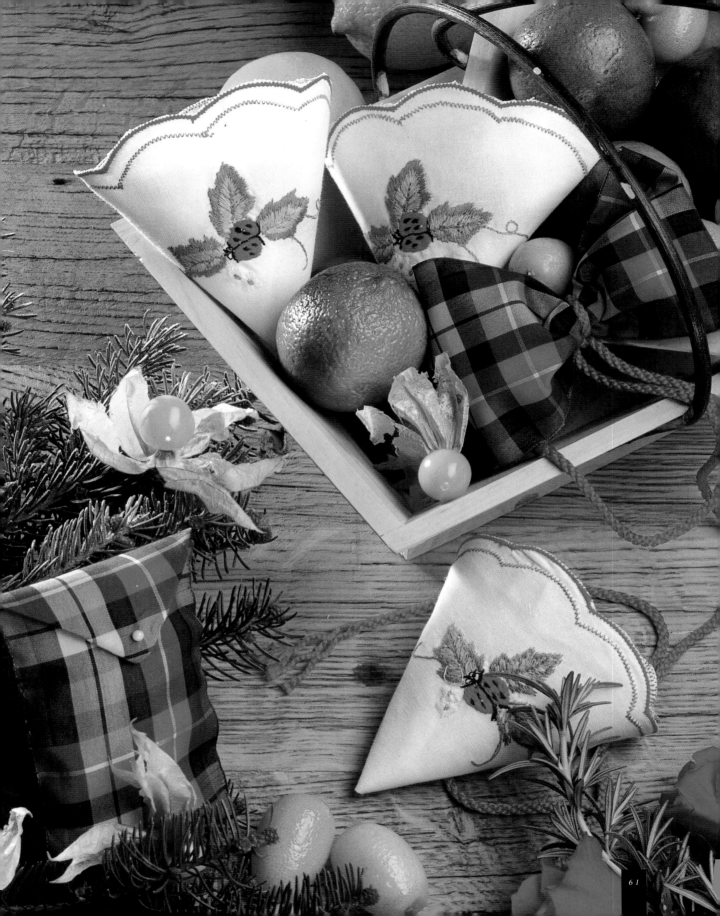

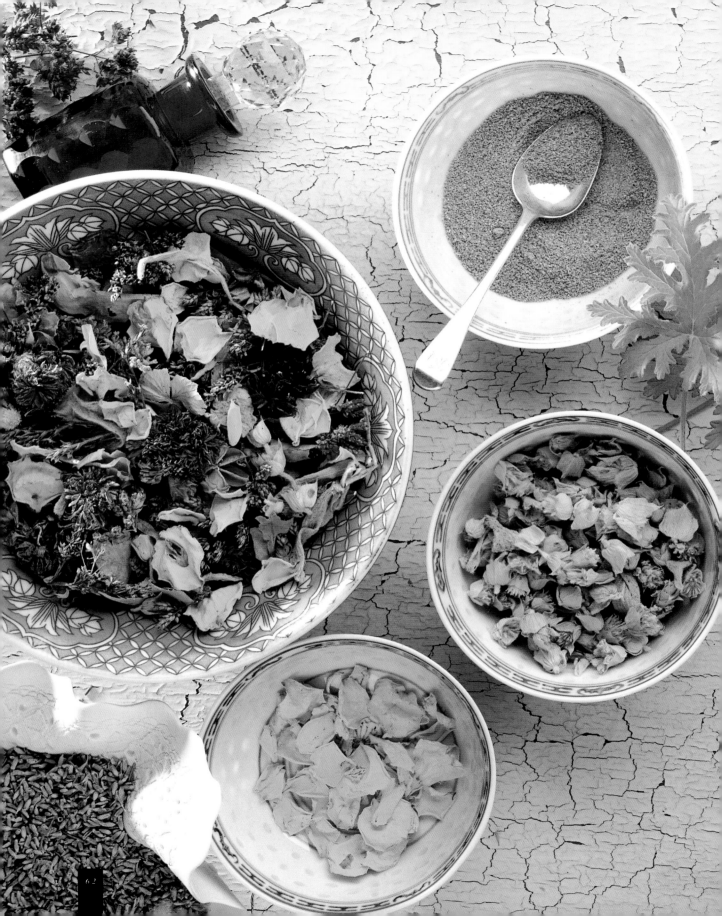

Perfumed Pot-pourri

MAKING POT-POURRI AT HOME is a great way of using up all sorts of interesting petals, seedheads, buds, and leaves that have been collected from the yard or the countryside during the summer months.

An easy way of drying plant materials is to lay them on trays lined with sheets of newspaper, and slide them under a bed or a chest of drawers away from the light. After a few weeks, check that the items are all dry and brittle, and then seal them in plastic bags for later use.

Turn to pages 64–5 for our seasonal pot-pourri recipes. Many plants retain their scent even when they are dried, although essential oils can also be added to make the pot-pourri more fragrant. Many traditional pot-pourri mixtures are based on lavender and rose petals (see the Traditional Blend). However, you can reflect your individuality in your choice of plant materials, and other decorative additions such as shells, pebbles or glass beads.

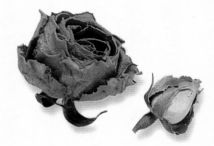

METHOD

Making a quick and easy dry pot-pourri:

✳ *Measure out and blend the essential oils into a small glass bottle — up to 100 drops of essential oil to every 8 cups/4oz (100g) of dry plant materials. Put the lid on and set it to one side.*

✳ *Grind all the powdered materials and the fixative (orris root powder) together with a pestle and mortar. Add half the total quantity of essential oils to this and mix.*

✳ *Put the main carrier ingredients of the pot-pourri into a storage container (such as a large jar), add the rest of the essential oil blend, and mix well.*

✳ *Gently mix in the powdered materials.*

✳ *Set aside a few decorative pot-pourri ingredients.*

✳ *Finally, seal the container and leave in a dark place to mature for between two and six weeks*

✳ *Display in a wide ceramic bowl or glass dish, arranging the decorative ingredients or other attractive items carefully on top.*

✳ *Alternatively, pack the pot-pourri into clear cellophane bags and seal with a decorative ribbon to present as a gift. Pot-pourri can also make a decorative base for presenting other presents such as soap, bath bags, or massage oils.*

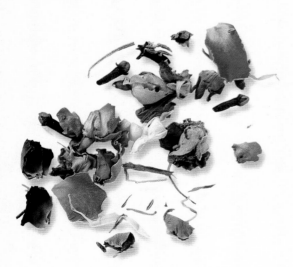

Pot-pourri Recipes

TRADITIONAL BLEND

2 cups/1oz (25g) dried mixed rose petals

1 cup/½oz (12g) dried verbena leaves

½ cup/¼oz (6g) dried lavender flowers

½ cup/¼oz (6g) dried mint leaves

½ tblsp orris root powder

Half a nutmeg, grated

20-25 drops rose essential oil

20-25 drops lavender essential oil

Decorative rosebuds

SUNSET BLUE

2 cups/1oz (25g) yellow rose petals and buds

1 cup/½oz (12g) dried delphinium flowers

1 cup/½oz (12g) dried marjoram flowers

1 cup/½oz (12g) dried blue hydrangea florets

1 cup/½oz (12g) dried scented geranium leaves

1 cup/½oz (12g) dried larkspur flowers

1 cup/½oz (12g) dried cornflowers

1 cup/½oz (12g) tiny sprays of dried blue sea lavender

1 cup/½oz (12g) dried chamomile flowers

1 cup/½oz (12g) dried lavender flowers

1 cup/½oz (12g) dried eucalyptus leaves, crumbled

½ tblsp orris root powder, ½ tblsp cumin powder

10 drops oakmoss essential oil, 10 drops cypress essential oil

20 drops rose essential oil

10 drops black pepper essential oil

CHRISTMAS SPICE

2 cups/1oz (25g) dried pink rose petals and buds

½ cup/¼oz (6g) dried bay leaves, crumbled

½ cup/¼oz (6g) dried orange peel

½ cup/¼oz (6g) dried pomegranate slices, chopped

1 tblsp grated nutmeg, ½ cup/¼oz (6g) small pine cones

½ tblsp orris root powder, 1 tsp cinnamon powder

½ tsp mixed spices, lightly crushed: mustard seed, black, green and white peppercorns, red spindle berries, juniper berries

10 drops frankincense essential oil, 5 drops clove essential oil

20 drops orange essential oil, 5 drops myrrh essential oil

ORIENTAL BREEZE

2 cups/1oz (25g) dried pink rose petals and buds

1 cup/½oz (12g) dried lavender heads

½ cup/¼oz (6g) star anise

½ cup/¼oz (6g) dried honesty seed heads

½ tblsp orris root powder

½ tblsp whole cloves (crushed)

10 drops sandalwood essential oil

5 drops geranium essential oil

10 drops jasmine essential oil

20 drops lavender essential oil

5 drops vanilla essential oil

Pictured: Christmas Spice pot-pourri.

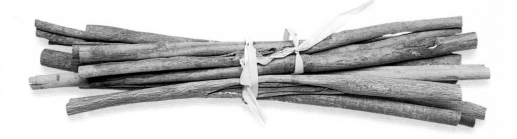

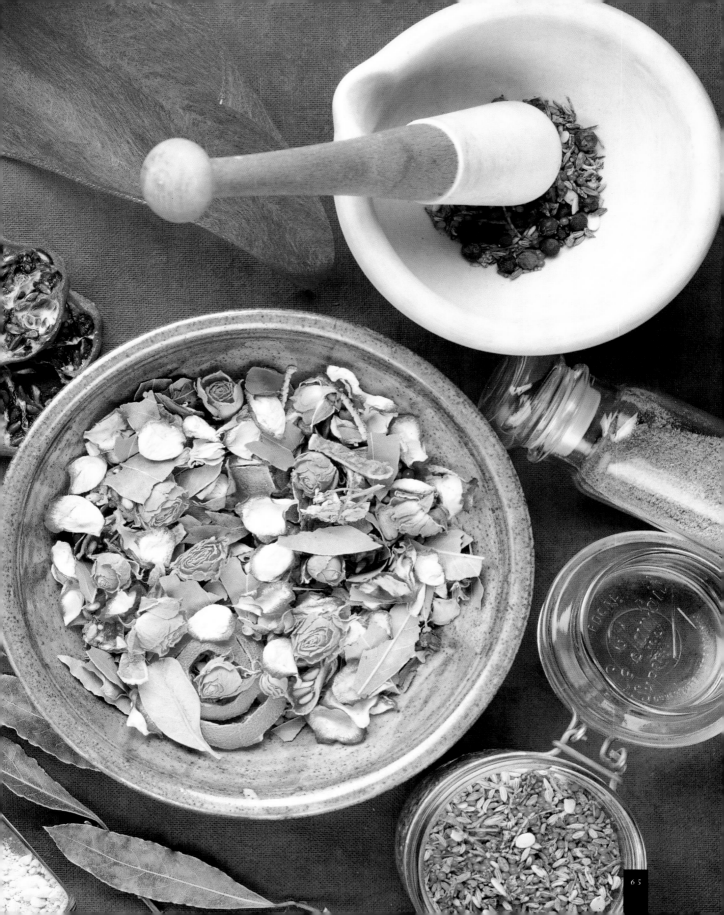

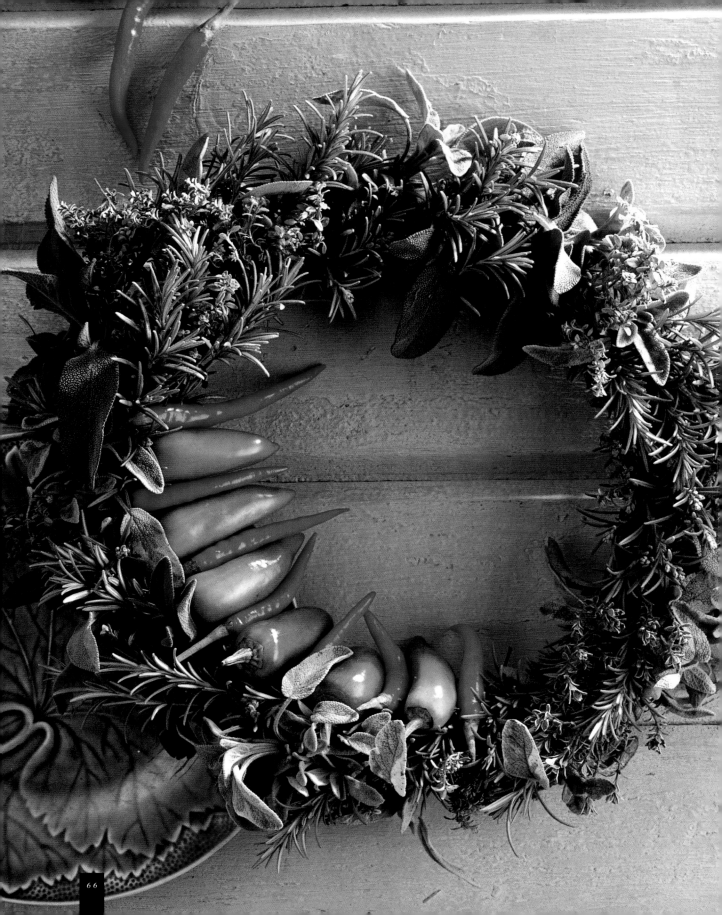

A Herb And Spice Ring

PEOPLE HAVE MADE SCENTED GARLANDS and evergreen wreaths for winter decorations for centuries, and they are still an important part of our Christmas celebrations. However, it is also possible for a beautiful plant-based arrangement to be useful as well as decorative.

An original gift, which will be much appreciated by those who love cooking, is to prepare a garland using materials which are invaluable to a well-stocked kitchen. Just as onions look more appealing when they are dangling from rustic strings, so herbs and spices come to life when they are displayed in the form of a herb or spice ring. Dried garlic, chillies or a mixture of bouquet garni herbs look very effective when they are used individually to make a

YOU WILL NEED

8 lengths of dried willow or a 8in (20cm) narrow twig ring (from florists)

6-8 red chilli peppers, 6-8 green chilli peppers

Fresh rosemary, Fresh sage (variegated and purple)

Fresh thyme (lemon scented and "Silver Posie")

Fine, medium-gauge and heavy-gauge floristry wire

Decorative ribbon

METHOD

✳ *Make a base by twisting the willow together into a circle. Bind it with heavy-gauge wire. Fix a decorative ribbon to the base to hang it with.*

✳ *Trim the herbs and arrange them into small bunches, securing each bunch with fine wire. Each bunch should contain rosemary, and one or other of the thymes and sages.*

✳ *Start to attach the bunches to the base, using short lengths of fine wire, laying each bunch so it overlaps the previous one and conceals any wiring.*

✳ *Thread alternate red and green chillies on to medium-gauge wire, and twist the ends into the ring so the spices form an arc at the top.*

garland. Alternatively, a mixture of useful culinary spices and herbs can be bound together to create a more elaborate circlet, which can be hung on a kitchen wall.

Our colorful herb and spice ring will emit a delightful fresh, herby fragrance.

Aromatic Bath Kits

THE THERAPEUTIC EFFECTS of aromatic bathing have been recognized for centuries. Roman bath houses, along with hot and cold baths and steam rooms, had a room for fragrant massage treatments, known as the unctuarium.

One of the easiest and most popular ways of creating a scented bath is to add between 5 and 10 drops of an essential oil (or a blend of oils) to the water. A selection of essential oils presented on a bed of pot-pourri makes an entrancing Christmas gift. For a sporty selection, include lavender for aches and pains, rosemary as an invigorating tonic, and marjoram for soothing tired muscles. For a sensual selection, choose rose, ylang ylang and sandalwood; a relaxing kit might comprise lavender, chamomile, and clary sage.

Essential oils can also be mixed with a vegetable oil base, such as jojoba, before being added to the bath. This helps to moisturise the skin and ensures an even distribution of the essential oils. Use the following relaxing blend as a guide:

METHOD

✤ *Mix the essential oils with the jojoba oil. (Jojoba has the advantage of not going rancid even if it is kept for some time.) Pour into a decorative tinted glass bottle.*

✤ *Tie a ribbon around the neck of the bottle, together with a tag giving instructions for use — "add a teaspoonful of this mixture to the bathwater before bathing."*

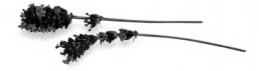

YOU WILL NEED

200 drops essential oils (50 drops clary sage, 50 drops roman chamomile, 100 drops lavender)

⅔ cup/¼pt (150ml) jojoba oil

Tinted bottles, Ribbon

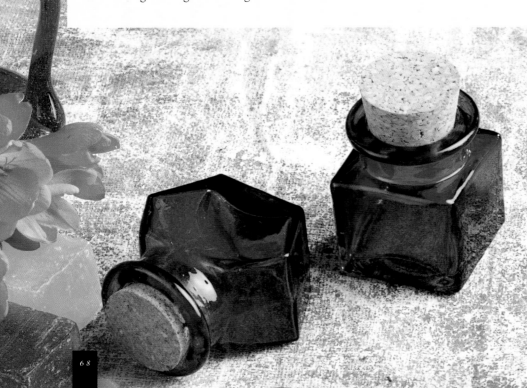

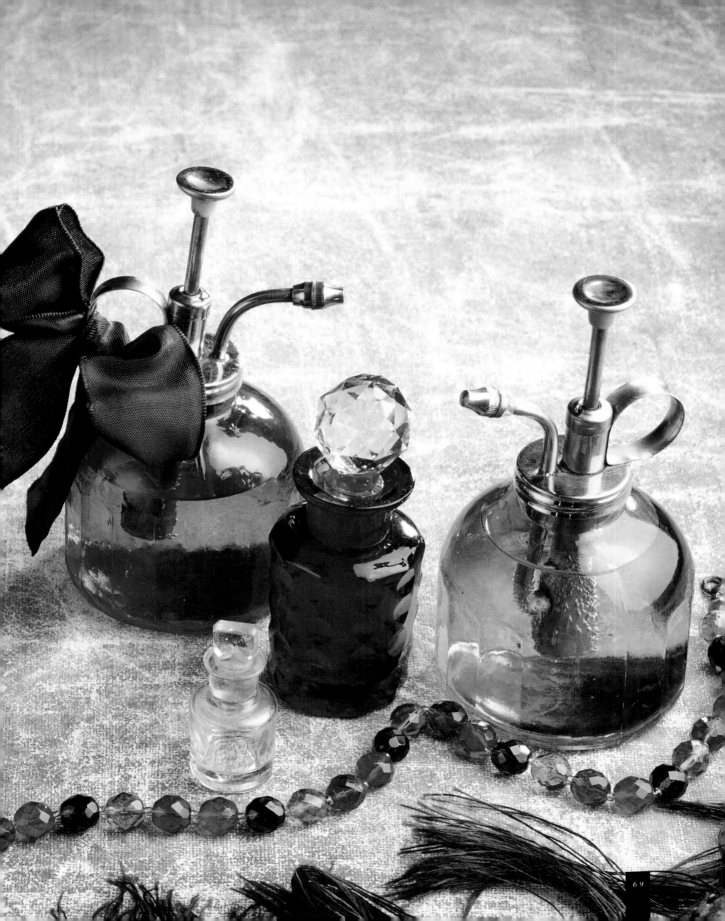

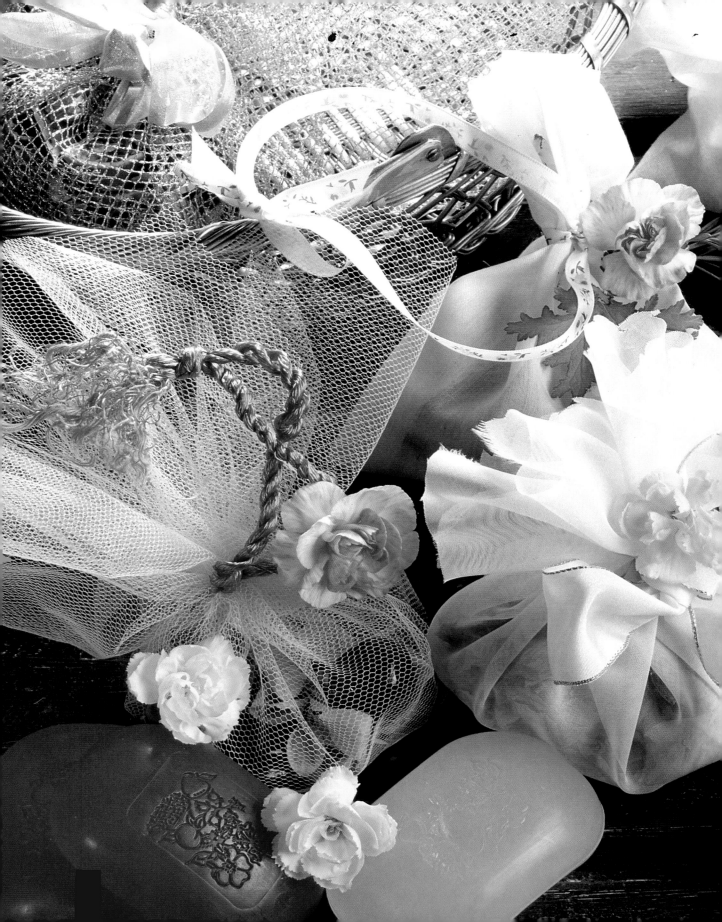

Bath Sacs

ANOTHER TRADITIONAL WAY of scenting the bath is to gather together a selection of fresh and dried herbs such as rosemary sprigs, dried lemon balm or lemon verbena leaves. Tie them together in a muslin bag with a piece of string or ribbon. Choose herbs both for their therapeutic properties and for their scent. Our herbal selection helps promote physical and mental relaxation.

YOU WILL NEED

Handful of dried lavender heads

Handful of dried chamomile flowers

Handful of dried lemon verbena leaves

Handful of dried lemon balm leaves

Small pieces of muslin and cotton net

Decorative ribbons and cords

METHOD

✳ *Mix the herbs together. If required, add a few drops of a chosen essential oil to the mixture to enhance the fragrance.*

✳ *Cut out a 12in (30cm) square of fabric. Put a heap of herbs in the middle and draw into a sac. Tie the neck with cord or ribbon.*

✳ *For an alternative sac, cut a strip of fabric 12in x 6in (30cm x 15cm). Cut the ends into a zigzag pattern if desired. Fold the cloth in half and sew the two side edges together, leaving the top open so it forms a small sac. Turn the sac inside out so the seams are concealed on the inside. Fill with herbs and tie with ribbon.*

✳ *To use the bath sac, tie it to the faucet by its ribbon, so it hangs in a stream of hot water while the bath is running.*

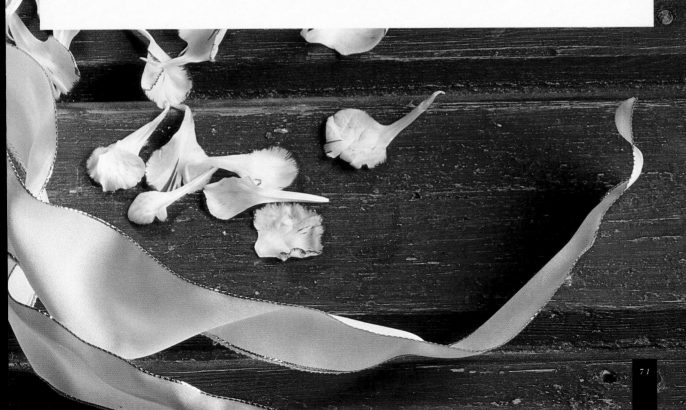

Fragrant Massage Oils

A MASSAGE OR BODY OIL is best applied to the body after bathing, when the pores of the skin are still open. Before being applied to the skin, essential oils are always diluted in a carrier oil, usually a light vegetable oil such as sweet almond or grapeseed.

When preparing a massage or body oil, the proportion of the essential oil to the carrier oil should be between 0.5% and 3%, depending upon the type of essential oil and intended therapeutic purpose. For general massage, a 2.5% dilution is suitable for adults. Body oils for those with sensitive skin, and facial lotions, should be even more dilute (0.5-1%). Babies, children and pregnant women also require very dilute blends (0.5%).

HOW MUCH ESSENTIAL OIL DO I NEED?

For 50ml (3 tblsp) carrier oil:

Blend percentage	Essential oil in drops
0.5%	5
1%	10
1.5%	15
2%	20
2.5%	25
3%	30

The shelf life of a blended massage or body oil is up to three months if 5-15% of wheatgerm oil is included in the vegetable oil base. A more stable carrier is jojoba oil, a liquid wax which does not go rancid. The essential oils themselves will begin to oxidize as soon as they come into contact with the carrier oil.

YOU WILL NEED

2 tblsp jojoba oil
(or sweet almond oil or grapeseed oil)

1 tblsp wheatgerm oil

1 tblsp rosehip oil

3-5 drops lavender essential oil

3-5 drops neroli (or petitgrain) essential oil

3-5 drops frankincense essential oil

METHOD

❋ Pour jojoba oil into a dark glass bottle. Use glass, not plastic, as this will help to preserve it for longer. (Jojoba is especially suited to those with dry or mature skin, sweet almond oil is good for normal or combination skin, and grapeseed oil benefits oily or blemished complexions.) Add the wheatgerm and rosehip oils.

❋ Add the essential oils and shake gently. To present as a gift, tie a ribbon with a tag (stating the ingredients) around the neck of the bottle, and bed it in a small basket filled with pot-pourri.

The basic recipe detailed here is a good, general-purpose body or massage oil. You can use it to soothe the body and emotions, and revitalize the skin. You might like to add a few massage tips to the bottle's tag, if you're giving the oil as a gift.

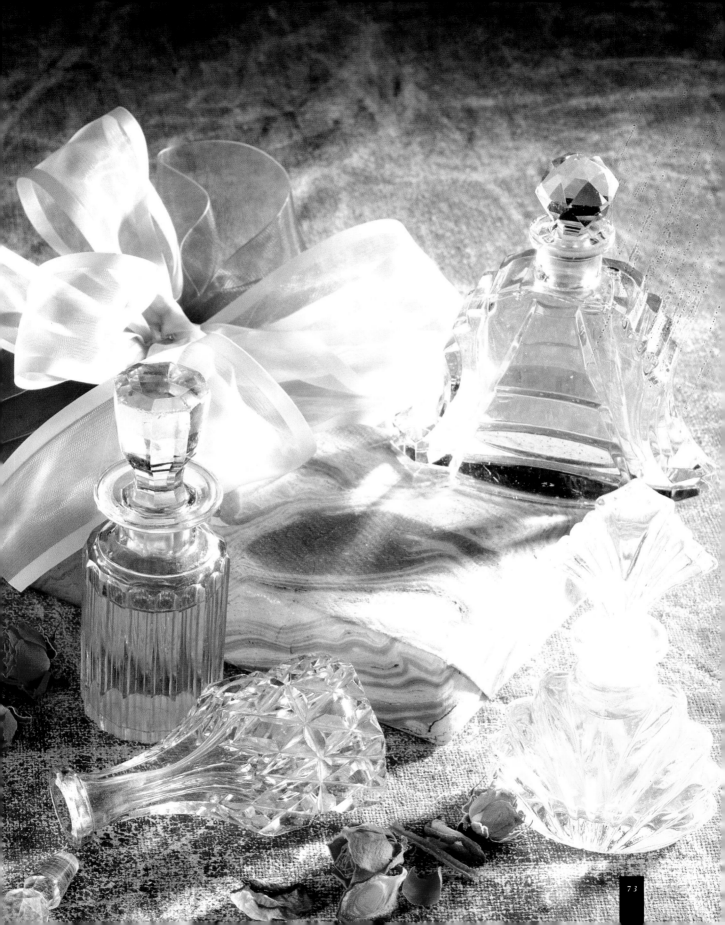

Light Perfumes

PERFUME IS ONE of the most popular Christmas gifts. Today most perfumes are made almost entirely from synthetic chemicals, rather than from pure essential oils or resins derived from plants, as they were originally.

Producing a sophisticated and concentrated natural perfume at home requires training and dedication. However, it is possible to make all kinds of light "aqua-based" fragrances with a minimum of expertise. These will be pleasant to use, although they will be lighter and less strongly fragranced than traditional, store-bought perfumes. You must use some kind of light or unscented diluting liquid as the base.

YOU WILL NEED

EAU-DE-PORTUGAL TOILET WATER

20 drops sweet orange oil

5 drops bergamot oil , 2 drops lemon oil

2 drops benzoin oil , I drop geranium oil

I tblsp vodka, 150ml (¼pt /⅔ cup) spring water

Coffee filter papers

METHOD

❋ *Dissolve the oils in the vodka. Add to the water, shaking well.*

❋ *Leave to mature for at least a month, then filter. Package in an attractive bottle with a decorative handwritten label.*

It is easy to make flower waters, which are beneficial for all types of skin. Simply add 10-30 drops of essential oil (or a blend such as 10 drops each of lavender, rosemary and petitgrain) to ⅔ cup / ¼ pt (150ml) of spring water. Leave it to stand for up to a month, and then filter it using a coffee filter paper. (A more basic preparation can be made without filtering, but this will then require shaking before use.) These delicately scented waters can be used to perfume, freshen and hydrate the skin.

A variety of essential oils can be diluted with alcohol (or cider vinegar or witch hazel) to make toilet water, eau-de-Cologne or after-shave lotion. Experiment with various scents to find your favorite.

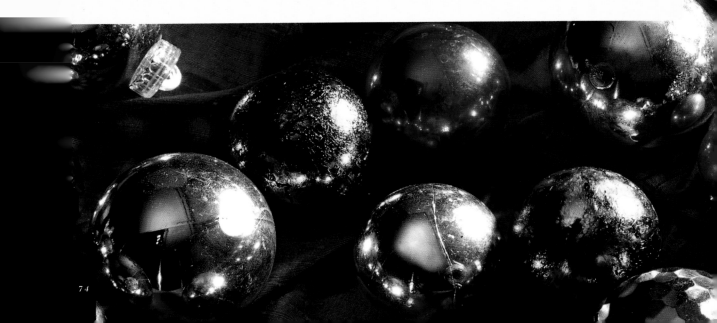

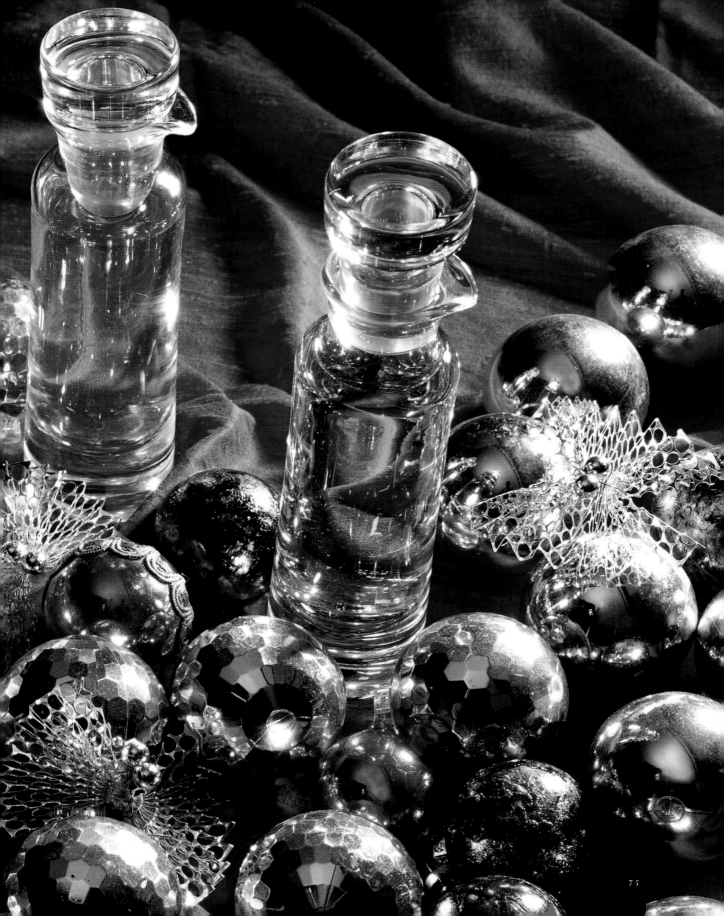

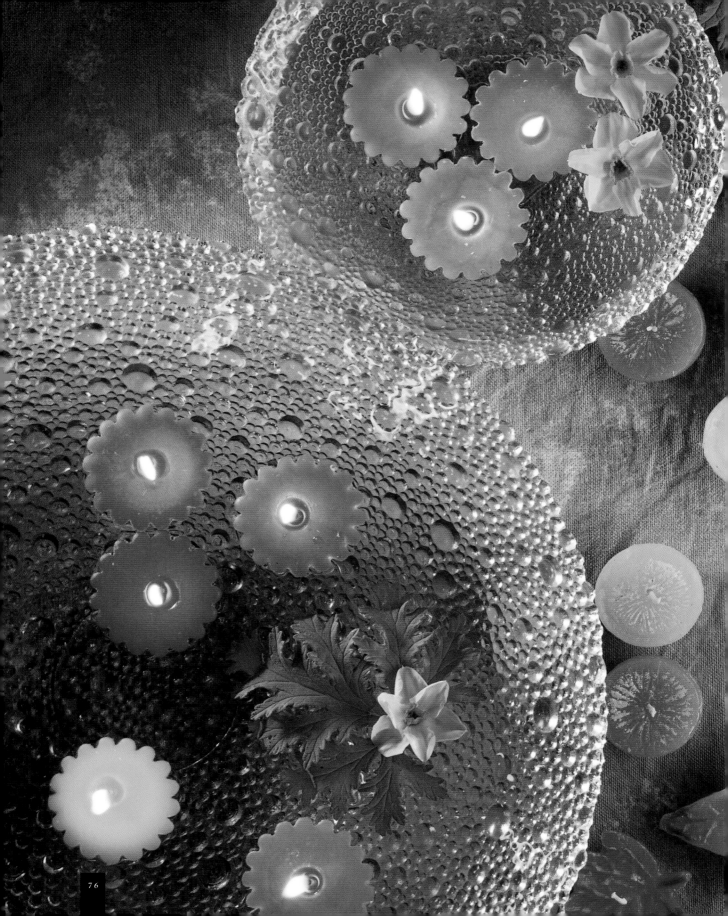

Scented Floating Candles

CANDLES ARE AN INTRINSIC PART of Christmas celebrations. Beeswax was one of the earliest materials used for candles, and it is still an excellent choice because it burns slowly and evenly whilst giving off a faint, honey scent. Church candles have always been made from beeswax, although it is more expensive than the paraffin wax which is now used for commercial candle-making.

The first American settlers made everyday candles from a native shrubby plant known as the wax myrtle, but for the Christmas festivities, they used wax from the bayberry. This plant was held in such high esteem that there were penalties for those who picked it before the given harvesting time.

The materials required for making candles at home can be found in specialist shops, but it is also worth remembering that old candle stubs can be recycled by melting them down in an old saucepan.

YOU WILL NEED

6oz (175g) natural beeswax
(or melted-down candle stubs)

30 drops of essential oils (10 drops each of myrtle, geranium and lavender makes a soothing, uplifting blend)

Candle wicks

Molds: scalloped metal cake or bun molds, flexible plastic leaf molds, eggshell halves

METHOD

✳ Melt the wax slowly in an old saucepan or a double boiler (a heatproof bowl over a pan of boiling water). Remove from the heat. Add the essential oils and mix gently, being careful to avoid introducing any air bubbles.

✳ Secure the wick to the base of the mold, using glue or a specialist wick holder. Pour the molten wax into the mold, keeping the wick upright. Leave the candle to set, then remove it from the mold.

✳ We made scalloped and leaf candles in purchased molds. We also improvised with half eggshells to make rounded candles. These had a pattern scratched into the wax before it had set completely.

✳ Float the candles in a decorative bowl of water.

✳ Never leave burning candles unattended.

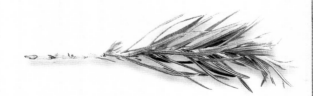

A Picture With A Difference

NATURAL FORMS — the colors of a fall leaf, the texture of a seashell or the pure aromatic appeal of a fragrant flower — have a simple beauty. Gifts made from them have an enduring quality. "Found" objects, such as a piece of driftwood encountered on a lonely beach, or flowers picked during a walk in the countryside, will carry the memory of the moment with them.

There are all sorts of ways of using natural forms for craftwork: some very traditional, such as pressing flowers or leaves to make pictures, and some more innovatory, such as making unique collages of "found" items. Many household objects can be decorated with pebbles, shells, leaves or pressed flowers. A plain mirror edged, for example, with a border of dried star anise, or a small box sprayed gold then decorated with pressed bay leaves,

---

YOU WILL NEED

Small picture frame made of driftwood

Shells, Essential oil

Handmade paper, Glue

Dried pressed herbs, such as lavender,
or marigold heads

METHOD

❋ Cut the handmade paper to fit the frame. Starting in the middle of the paper, glue the dried pressed herbs in place in an attractive design. If you wish, the paper can then be scented. Place it in a sealed container for a week with a cotton pad soaked in a few drops of essential oil.

❋ (The shells may also be scented before use by placing in a jar for a week with a few drops of essential oil.) Glue the shells to the driftwood frame. Insert your herb paper into the frame.

❋ It is also fun and easy to make your own handmade paper, to which small pieces of leaf or flower can be added during the process. There are many craft books on the subject. Additionally, handmade paper can be scented by adding a few drops of essential oil to the wet paper pulp mix.

are lovely, easy-to-make gifts. Our scented picture draws on the different shapes and textures found in nature. Use our suggestions to inspire you to create your own, unique picture.

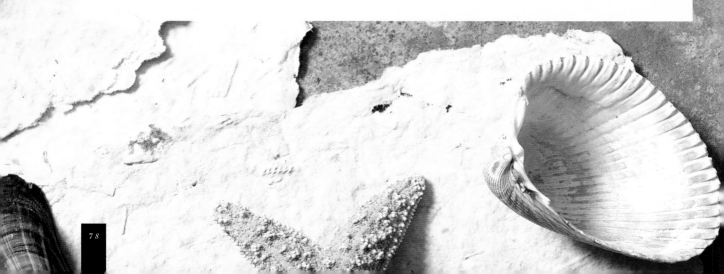

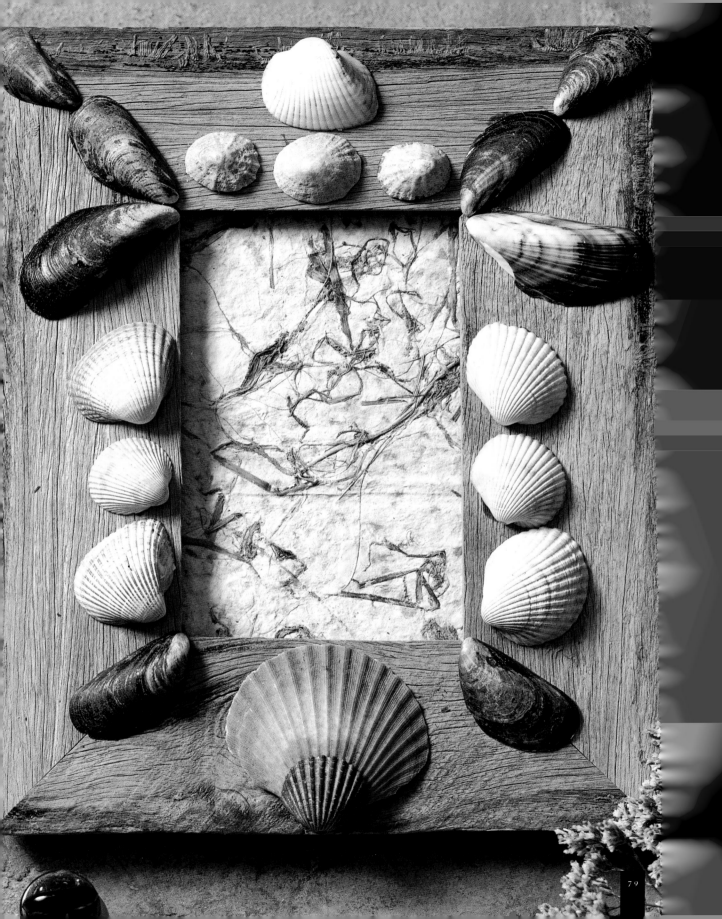

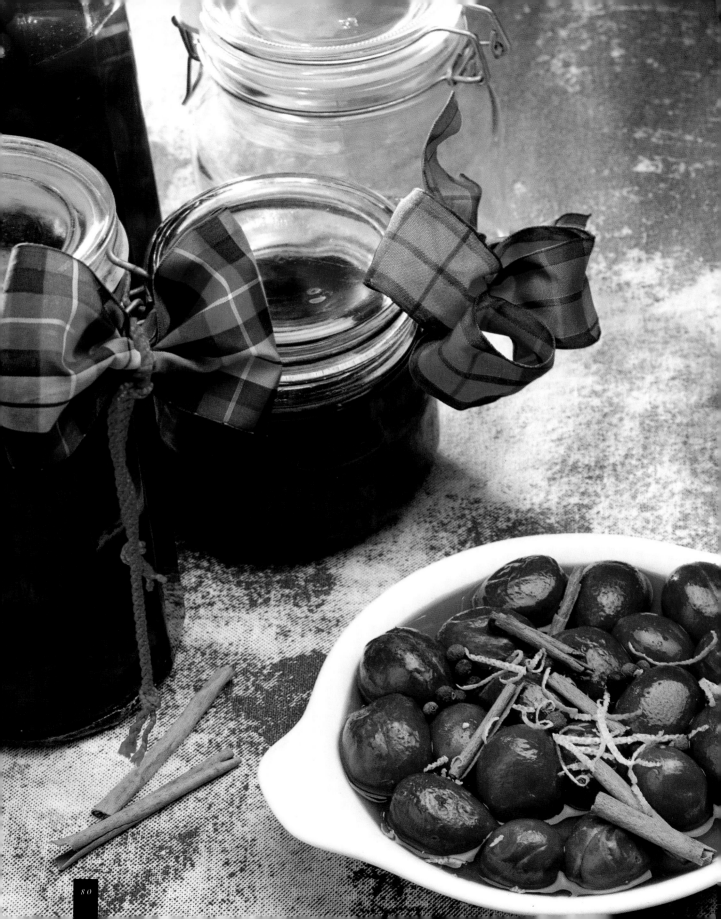

Spiced Plums

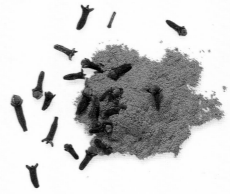

THE USE OF AROMATIC SPICES was widespread in England in the seventeenth to nineteenth centuries. Sweet dishes and cakes were full of nutmeg, mace, cinnamon and cloves. Nutmeg was so popular that fastidious travelers always carried a small nutmeg with them, encased in small silver pocket graters complete with compartments for the nut.

All spices are best stored whole in an airtight container, as they lose aroma and flavor quickly once ground. Mace comes from the outer covering of the nutmeg, and has a similar, though stronger and more pungent flavor. Cinnamon was an essential ingredient in medieval cookery, particularly popular in France. Today, it is used in desserts and meat dishes. It is also an essential ingredient of mulled wine and spiced ales.

Cloves were referred to as "grains of paradise" in medieval French recipes, and used lavishly, particularly by the aristocracy. Allspice, or Jamaica pepper, has a fragrant aroma similar to cloves, but tastes like a mixture of cinnamon, nutmeg, and cloves. Its aromatic qualities make it an essential ingredient in spicing or pickling mixtures, and equally popular for pot-pourri.

YOU WILL NEED

4lb (2 kg) plums

Grated rind and juice of I orange and I lemon

2 cups/1lb (450g) soft brown sugar (light brown sugar)

12 cloves, 2 cinnamon sticks

I tsp ground mace or nutmeg, 10 whole allspice

2½ cups/1pt (600ml) red wine vinegar

4 tbslp Drambuie liqueur

METHOD

✳ Wash the plums. Remove stalks, then partially split to remove the stones. Layer the plums in a casserole dish with the grated orange and lemon rind, and sugar. Sprinkle with orange and lemon juice, cover and leave overnight in a cool place.

✳ The next day, add cloves, cinnamon sticks, allspice and mace, distributing the spices evenly. Add the wine vinegar and Drambuie.

✳ Put on the casserole lid and bake the plums slowly at the bottom of the oven for four hours at 140°C / 275°F / Gas mark 1. Once cooked, leave to cool in the dish.

✳ Remove the cloves, cinnamon and allspice. Store the fruit in decorative jars, tightly covered with waxed paper. Make attractive handwritten labels.

✳ Leave the spiced plums for two to three months before eating. Spiced plums are delicious with cold meats and all kinds of game, including turkey.

Herbal Vinegars And Oils

ALMOST ALL CULINARY HERBS can be used to flavor vinegars and oils. They have been used in this way for centuries, especially in the Mediterranean region. Certain herbs are better suited to being steeped in either oil or vinegar, for use as a salad dressing or for specific cooking requirements. Herbs can also be blended to provide a range of flavors.

The principal herbs used for making herb vinegars are basil, bay, chervil, chives, dill, fennel, garlic, juniper, lavender, lovage, marjoram, mint, oregano, rosemary, sage, tarragon, and thyme.

The best herbs for flavoring olive oil are basil, bay, chervil, dill, fennel, garlic, juniper, lavender, lovage, marjoram, mint, parsley, rosemary, sage, savory, and thyme.

YOU WILL NEED
PROVENÇAL VINEGAR

1¼ cups/½pt (300ml) white wine vinegar

2-3 cloves of garlic (peeled)

Sprig each of fresh thyme and rosemary

METHOD

✳ *The method for making a herbal vinegar or oil could not be easier! Simply remove the lid from the bottle of white wine vinegar (or top-quality virgin olive oil) and add a few sprigs of your chosen herb to the bottle – for this recipe, thyme, rosemary, and garlic.*

✳ *Seal the bottle tightly, put it in a warm place and leave for one to two weeks until the essence of the herbs has been absorbed.*

✳ *When the vinegar or oil is to be presented as a gift, use a decorative airtight bottle. Tie a bright ribbon round the neck of the bottle, together with a label listing the aromatic ingredients. The bottle looks more attractive with the herbs still in it, but unless it is kept in a cool, dark place, these will gradually discolor. To avoid this, the herbs can be removed from the bottle after a few weeks.*

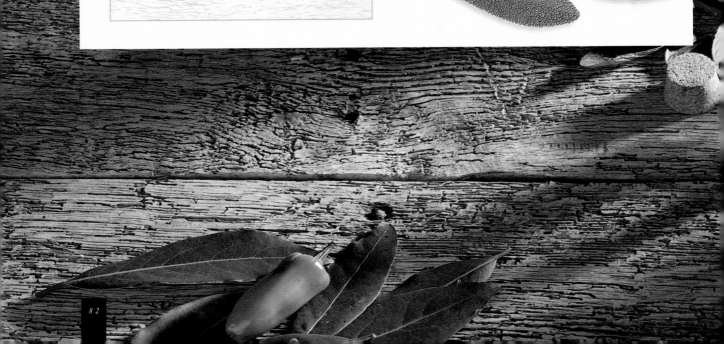

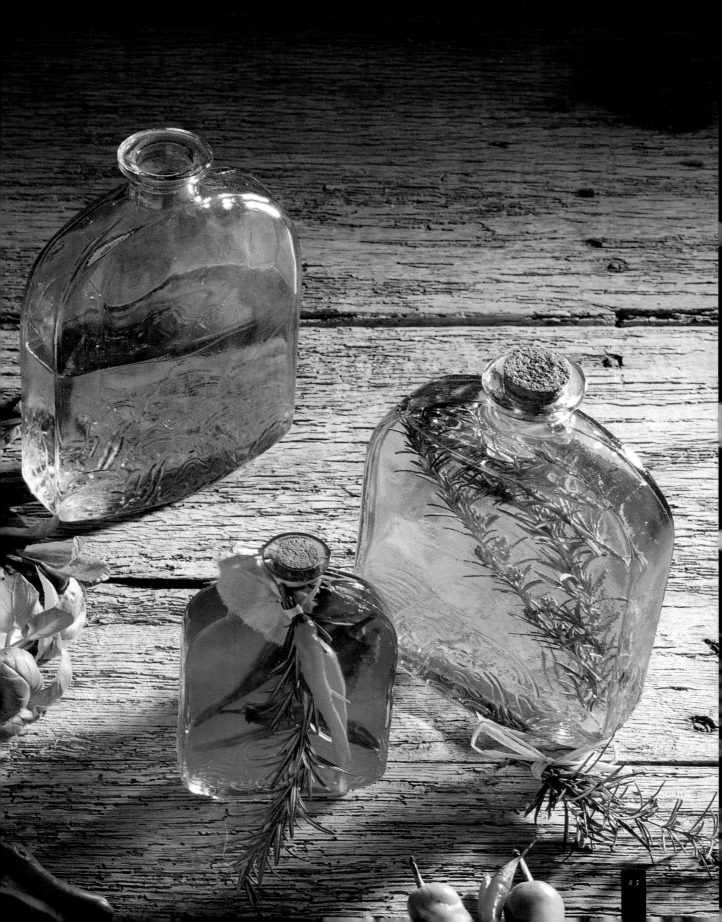

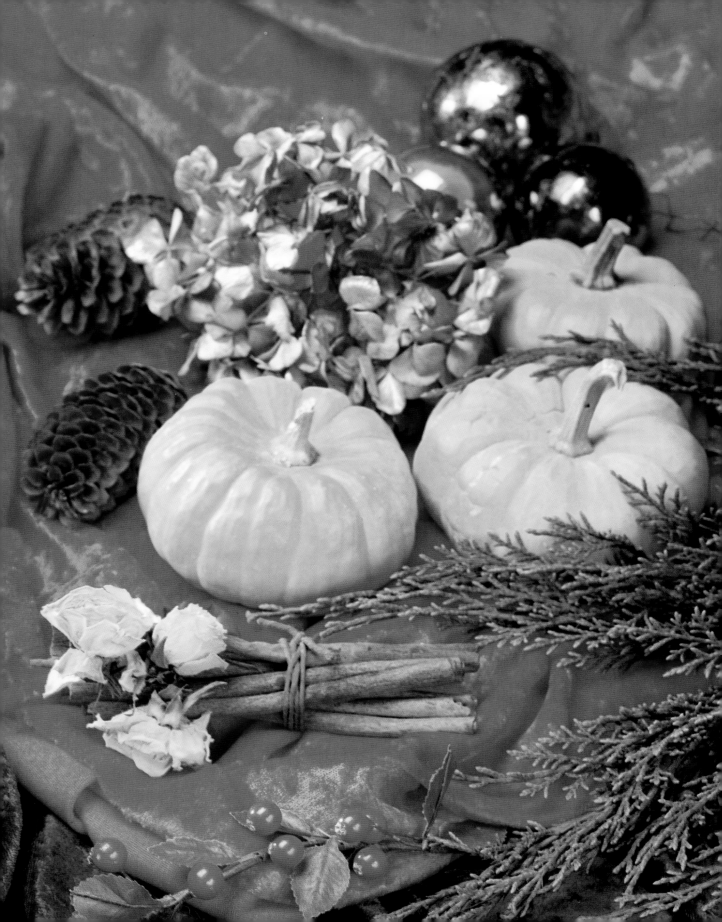

PART THREE

Seasonal Home Treats

A SCENTED HOME IS PARTICULARLY appreciated at Christmas, as it helps add to the festive atmosphere. Many decorative items can be perfumed, giving an extra dimension to their visual appeal. We have shown three ideas: a dried rose ball, miniature topiary tree, and perfumed Christmas stockings.

Miniature topiary "trees" can also be made from living plants for use indoors. Grow aromatic herbs in pots and clip them into simple shapes. Perennial herbs such as bay, lavender, rosemary, santolina, and scented geraniums all make good subjects for topiary, as they thrive on constant clipping and make well-shaped bushes. Since these herbs can easily be grown from cuttings, they also make delightful yet economical gifts, especially if the pots are decorated by hand with stencils or a simple floral design.

LEFT: Enrich your home with an array of bright colors.

RIGHT: Christmas can be made into a feast for all the senses.

AROMATIC RECIPES

Feasting is central to Christmas. Our sense of continuity and tradition is reflected in the food we eat, despite changes over the centuries and variations from country to country. Aromatic and sweet-smelling spices are found in most Christmas dishes and drinks, and echo the exotic spices of frankincense and myrrh brought to the Christ child by the Three Kings.

*"The wind is blowing coldly,
The night is dark and drear,
And we would gladly linger,
To taste your Christmas cheer."*

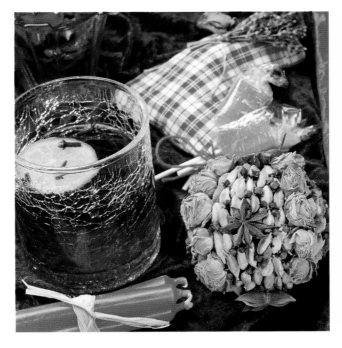

Certain fruits are popularly used in Christmas recipes because of their symbolic associations. Some examples are the apple, which symbolizes the Tree of Knowledge in Paradise; the orange, which is reminiscent of the sun; and nuts, with their hard shells and sweet kernels, which are symbolic of the simultaneous harshness and rewards of life. Communal feasting not only brings the year to a close with a sense of abundance, but also holds out the hope of a fruitful year to come.

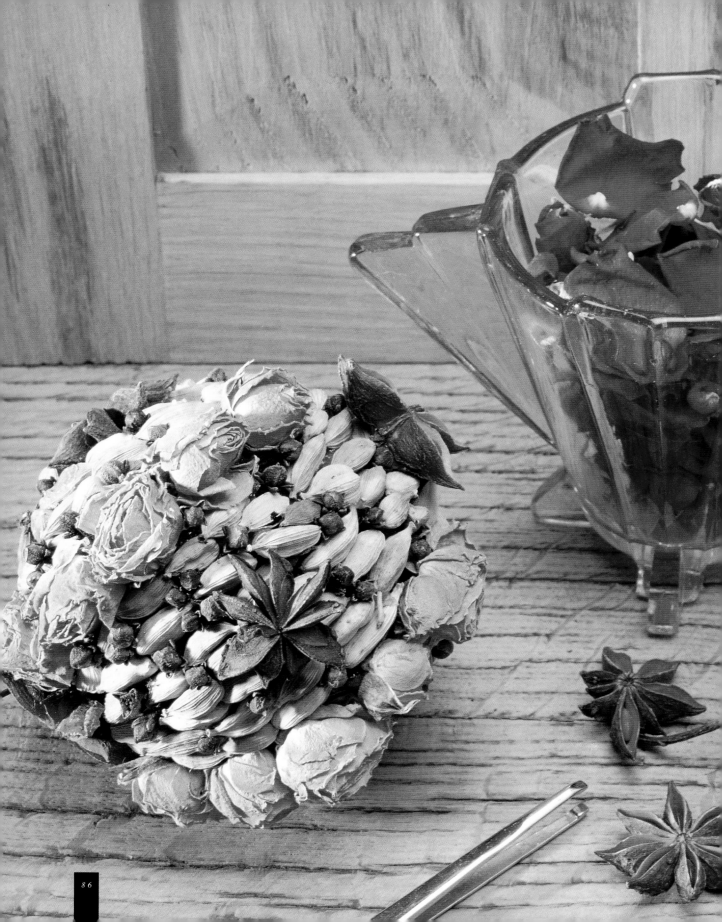

Dried Rose Ball

THE MOST DRAMATIC decorative effects can be achieved quite simply using floristry foam and a quantity of dried flower heads, herbs or evergreen foliage to create symmetrical or statuesque shapes. The compact, dried flower heads of plants such as lavender, statice, helichrysum, achillea or rosebuds are good for making long-lasting floral designs. Simple shapes are often the most attractive — spheres, cones or pyramids are the main traditional forms — although it is also possible to create a more elaborate design if you wish. The following instructions are for a hanging rosebud "spice ball."

YOU WILL NEED

Narrow decorative ribbon

Floristry foam ball, 7.5cm (3in) diameter

Floristry wire, Glue

3 handfuls of dried rosebuds

Handful of green cardamom pods

Handful of cloves, Dried star anise pods

Essential oils of rose and cardamom

METHOD

✳ Make a loop of the ribbon. Wrap one end of a piece of floristry wire securely around the loose ends of the ribbon, and push the other end of the wire through the centre of the foam ball and out the other side. Trim the wire to within 1in (3cm) of the ball, bend it back on itself, and push the end into the foam.

✳ Start to glue rows of rosebuds on to the foam ball, packing them closely together to create a dense effect.

✳ Fill the spaces between the rows with cardamom pods, cloves and star anise to add extra color and texture to the design. (Glue the cardamom and star anise; cloves can be pushed into the foam.)

✳ Finally, scent the completed ball with a few drops each of rose and cardamom essential oils. Cardamom oil is very powerful, so be careful not to use too many drops!

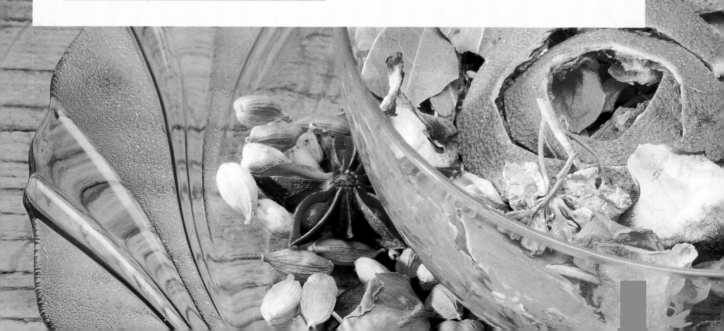

Miniature Topiary Trees

CREATE ARCHITECTURAL EFFECTS with evergreen foliage by turning it into miniature "trees" or "shrubs." Work it into the shape of a conical bay tree, a round box bush, or an open-branched magnolia. We have used fresh greenery, but you can make a longer-lasting tree by using dried evergreens such as moss, golden rod, box, juniper, or cypress for the "foliage." Flowers will add pretty highlights.

We have used a purchased twig ball on a ready-made stem, but you could also sculpt a square of floristry foam into the required shape. If the "foliage" is to sit on top of a short trunk, collect branches or twigs to achieve the desired effect. Alternatively, a round box ball looks very effective simply placed directly on top of a flowerpot.

YOU WILL NEED

Small terracotta pot

Twig ball on twisted twig stem (from florist's)

Plaster of paris, Slivers of foam, Gravel, Fresh box sprigs

Kumquats, Floristry stub wires

Juniper essential oil (or pine, cypress or cedarwood)

METHOD

✳ *Stand the box in water overnight to absorb as much moisture as possible (there is no moisture source in the twig ball).*

✳ *Line the terracotta pot with slivers of dry foam to prevent it from splitting as the plaster expands. Mix the plaster of paris to a smooth consistency and fill the pot up to a little below the rim. Quickly insert the base of the twig stem into the pot before the plaster starts to dry. Support the stem in an upright position until it stands up by itself. Leave the plaster to dry thoroughly.*

✳ *Carefully push the box sprigs into the twig ball until it is well covered.*

✳ *Wire the kumquats on to stub wires, and insert between the sprigs of box, securing them to the twig ball.*

✳ *Cover the top of the pot with gravel to conceal the plaster base. Finally, apply a few drops of a woody-scented essential oil to the whole arrangement to increase its aromatic appeal.*

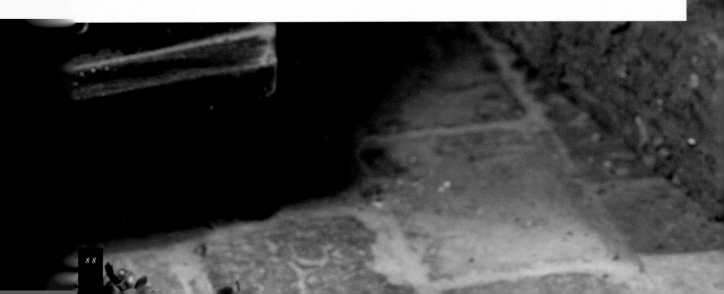

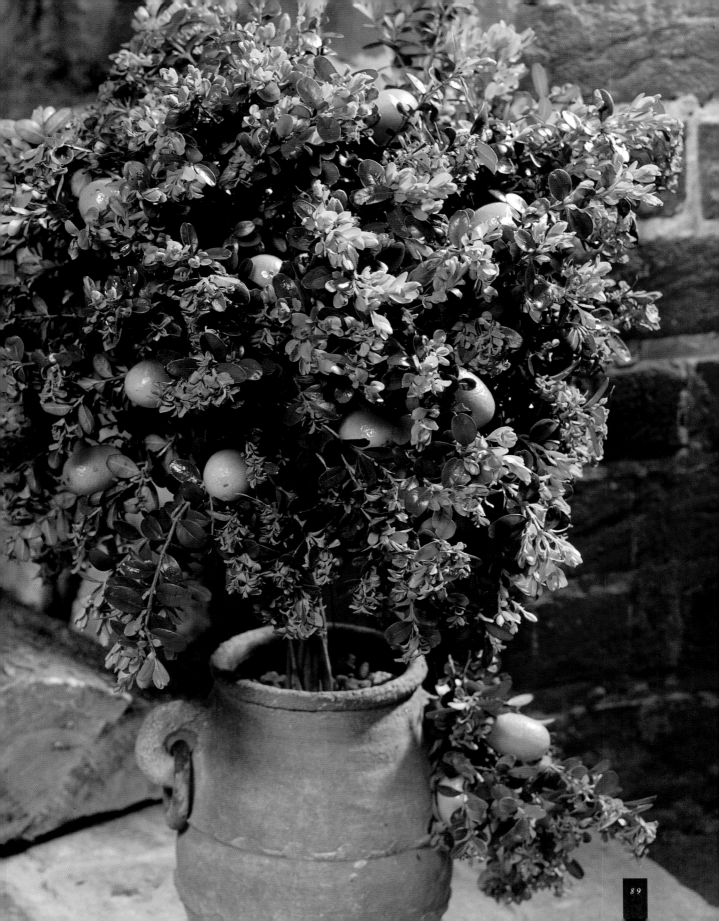

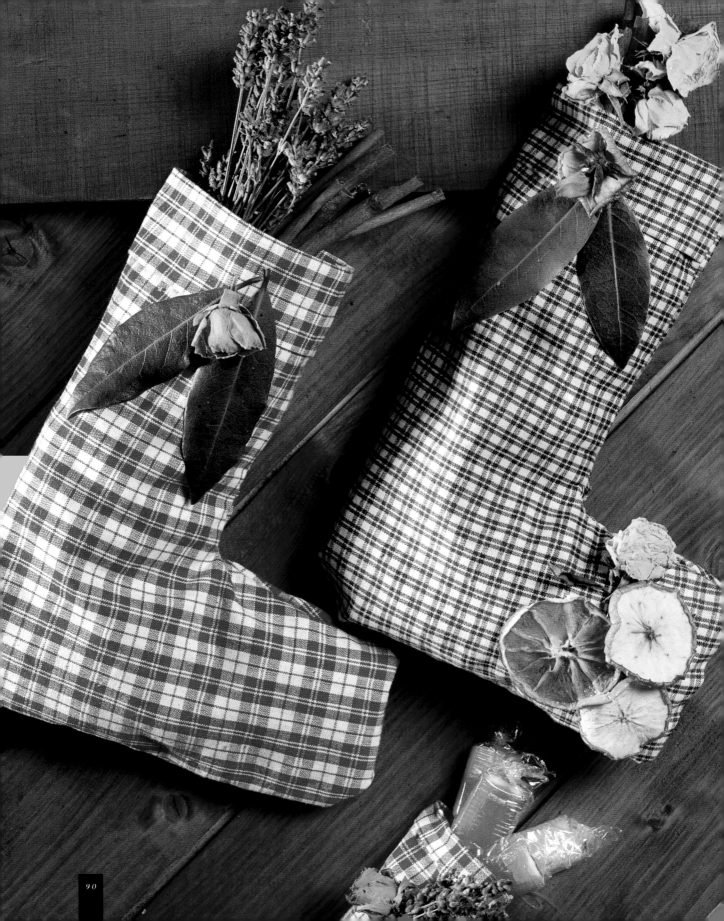

Perfumed Christmas Stockings

THESE CHARMING CHRISTMAS stocking decorations herald what, for children, is the most exciting part of the season – the Christmas Eve delivery of presents by Father Christmas. The figure of Father Christmas originated in pagan religion, as a friendly character who brought good cheer to people in the depths of winter.

Father Christmas is also known as Santa Claus or St. Nicholas, but this strand of the legend is based on history. St. Nicholas was one of the first bishops of the Christian Church, who later became the patron saint of children. On the saint's feast day, children were traditionally given presents if they had been good during the year.

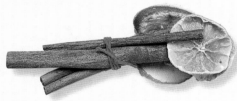

YOU WILL NEED

"Shaker" gingham in red and green

Dried apple and orange rings (see pages 30–1)

Dried lavender, Bay laurel leaves

Cinnamon sticks, Mini lollipops

Gold string, Essential oils (optional)

METHOD

✳ *Make paper patterns for the stockings. We made an assortment of sizes, for adults and children.*

✳ *Fold the fabric double, pin on the patterns, and cut out two pieces for each stocking.*

✳ *On the right side of each piece, fold over a small "cuff," tucking the raw edge under to neaten. Stitch this in place.*

✳ *With the right sides of the stocking together, sew from the top edge, down round the foot, and up to the opposite top edge. Leave the top open.*

✳ *Decorate the outside of the stockings by glueing on (or stitching) pieces of dried apple and orange, rosebuds, mini sprigs of lavender tied with gold string, and bay leaves.*

✳ *Fill the stockings. We used a bunch of dried lavender, dried rosebuds glued on to cinnamon sticks, and mini lollipops.*

✳ *If desired, all the dried plant materials can be given an extra boost of scent with a few drops of essential oil. The fabric for the stockings can also be pre-perfumed by enclosing in a sealed container with a pad imbued with a few drops of essential oil, for a week.*

Scented Circle Table Decoration

A DISPLAY OF FRESH FLOWERS and greenery adds life and color to the dining table, whatever the occasion. At Christmas, however, a sumptuous arrangement of aromatic plants enriches the festive spirit, especially when combined with candles and decorative tableware.

Decide on a theme for decorating the table, and match the colors of the candles, tablecloth and napkins to enhance the effect. Dark reds, purples and golds will create an exotic, oriental ambience; delicate pale green, silver and yellow give a lighter, softer touch to the table.

It is easy to make up an aromatic wreath (or a series of small circlets) based on scented evergreens, flowers and herbs for a table centerpiece. Individual circlets can also be joined together to form a chain. Follow our recommendations for plants, or substitute your own choice of greenery and flowers in season.

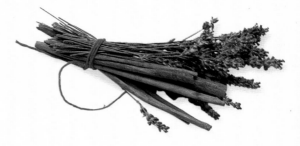

YOU WILL NEED

8in (20cm) floristry foam ring

Plastic ring holder

Greenery: sprigs of cypress, geranium,
scented geranium, rosemary, variegated sage
Flowers: freesias, pinks,
wax plant (Hoya carnosa), sea lavender,
12 taper candles

METHOD

❋ Soak the foam in cold water for a couple of hours, until it is saturated. Put it on some newspaper to absorb any excess water.

❋ Trim the plants to size. You can either use one type of greenery as the background, or you can create a more textured effect by interweaving a selection of leaf colors and shapes. Start to construct the background by arranging the greenery around the outside and inside of the ring, pushing each stem firmly into the foam.

❋ Slowly build up the ring with the rest of the greenery, keeping it as even and dense as possible. Add flowers to the arrangement to highlight its visual impact. Finally, insert the taper candles.

❋ Put the finished wreath in the plastic holder. This can be placed at the center of the table, or used to frame a candle or a plate of food.

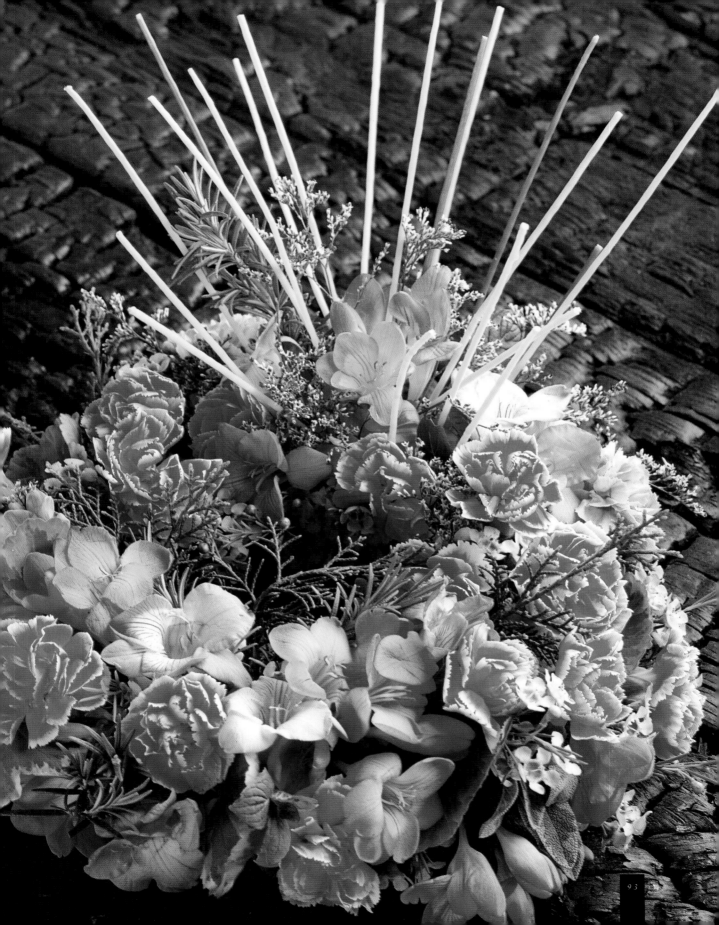

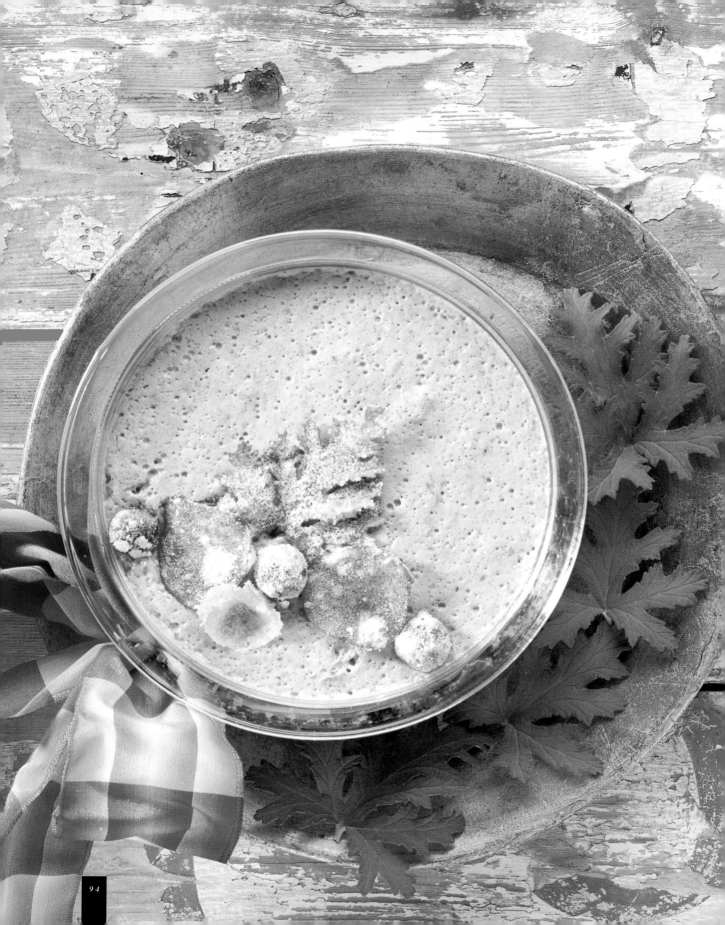

Frosted Fruit And Flowers

A DELIGHTFUL WAY of adding color and finesse to Christmas meals is to garnish food with a selection of frosted flowers, leaves and fruit. Frosted flowers were particularly popular during the Elizabethan age in England, when they were eaten as elegant after-dinner sweetmeats.

It is surprising how many flowers can be picked and eaten straight from the plant, providing they have not been sprayed with pesticides. Carnations, chrysanthemums, clover, cornflowers, cowslips, dahlias, daisies, forget-me-nots, hollyhocks, honeysuckle, hop flowers, jasmine, lilac, mallow, marigolds, nasturtiums, heartsease pansies, pinks, roses and violets are all edible. Although most of these plants are dormant in the middle of winter, some are available from florists' shops.

YOU WILL NEED

Egg white

Caster sugar (granulated sugar)

Crimson and scarlet rose petals

Scented geranium leaves

Primroses, Black grapes

METHOD

✳ Lightly whisk the egg white, then brush it on to all surfaces of the flower heads, leaves, petals and grapes.

✳ Dust each item lightly with sugar, shaking it gently to remove any excess. Place the coated items on a sheet of baking parchment on a wire rack, and leave in a warm place for several hours until completely dry.

✳ Although frosted flowers taste best when they have been freshly prepared, they can be stored for several months if kept in an airtight container (because the sugar acts as a preservative). The fruit is best eaten the same day.

✳ Use frosted flowers over the Christmas period for decorating all kinds of dishes, especially desserts such as ice-cream, sorbet, or cake.

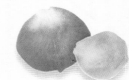

PICTURED: raspberry mousse with frosted fruit and flowers.

Napkin Decorations

IT IS WELL KNOWN that a few fresh green leaves can enhance the appeal of a dish – a sprig of fresh dill, fennel or basil is often used to garnish fish recipes. Herbs, however, can be used in all sorts of ways to provide contrast and interest. Shoots of rosemary, thyme, juniper, hyssop or bay can be tucked into napkins or used to decorate the plates of all the courses from the starters to the desserts. A ring of emerald mint leaves, for example, can be used to set off most sweet dishes. Flowering herbs are also valuable in this respect, not just for their delicate appearance, but for lightly flavoring salads and drinks. The flowers of borage, chamomile, chives, elderflower, hyssop, lavender, marjoram, mint, sage, tarragon, and thyme are especially suitable.

YOU WILL NEED

Cloth napkins (square and square with rounded corners)

Napkin rings, Scraps of silk, Decorative ribbons

Glue, Bay leaves, Rosemary, Scented geranium leaves

Freesias, Roses, Wax plant (Hoya carnosa)

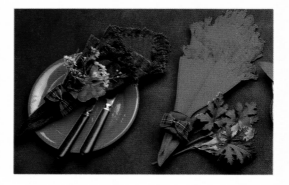

METHOD

❋ Cover the napkin rings with silk. Cut a rectangle the same length as the circumference of the napkin ring, plus turnings. (The width of the rectangle should be the same as the width of the napkin ring, plus turnings.) Stitch the ends of the silk together and turn the seam to the inside. Slip over the napkin ring. (For a more intricate pleated design, cut a longer rectangle, and pleat the cloth on to the

napkin ring.) Fold the silk over the sides of the napkin ring and glue in place. Create decorative bows out of the ribbon, and secure to the napkin ring with a couple of stitches.

❋ Fold the napkins with rounded corners into pocket shapes, as shown in the picture. Place a selection of the plants in the pocket.

❋ Fold the square napkins as shown in the picture above, and slip into the napkin rings. Push a few plants through the napkin rings.

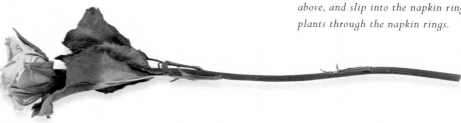

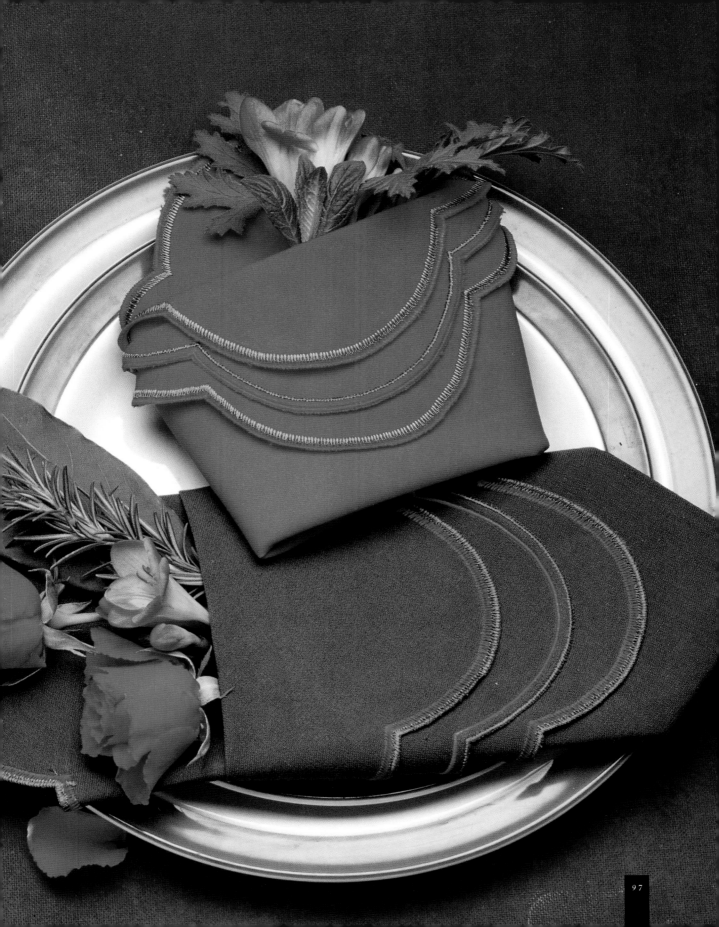

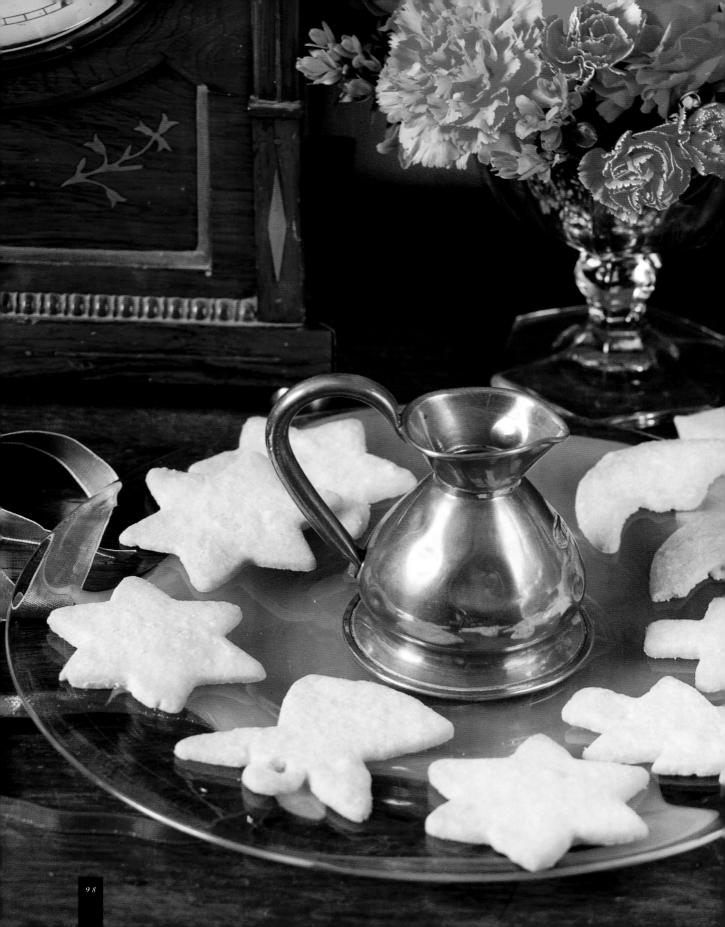

Advent Cookies

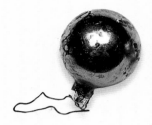
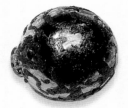

ADVENT, the period which includes the four Sundays before Christmas, marks the start of the festive season. In Scandinavian countries, Holland and Germany, it customary to serve an assortment of spiced, decorative cookies when family and friend gather together.

The feast of St. Nicholas falls on December 6th, and in Holland is celebrated on St. Nicholas' Eve, the evening of December 5th. This is the day when children receive their gifts and St. Nicholas appears in schools, throwing handfuls of sweets and small spiced cookies into the classrooms.

Our Advent cookies can be made in special wooden molds, or you can shape the cookie dough with a cookie cutter or by cutting out by hand. Make Christmas symbols such as trees and stars.

YOU WILL NEED

1lb (450g) plain flour, 1 tsp baking powder

¾ cup/10oz (275g) honey

⅔ cup/8oz (225g) golden syrup

¾ cup/6oz (175g) brown sugar

½ cup/4oz (100g) butter, Pinch of cardamom

1 tsp ground cinnamon, 1 tsp ground cloves

METHOD

✳ *Pre-heat the oven to 200°C/400°F/Gas mark 6. Melt the honey, golden syrup and sugar gently in a large saucepan over a moderate heat, stirring until the sugar is dissolved. Simmer on a low heat for 5 minutes. Slowly melt the butter into the mixture.*

✳ *In a separate bowl, mix together the flour, baking powder, cardamom, cloves and cinnamon.*

✳ *Take the pan off the stove and gradually blend in the flour and spice mixture.*

✳ *Once the batter is smoothly blended, pour into greased molds. Alternatively, cut out shapes and put on to a greased baking sheet, leaving 1in (2.5cm) between each cookie. (If you plan to hang the cookies on the Christmas tree, put a small hole in the top with a skewer before baking.) Bake for about 15 minutes, and then cool on a wire rack.*

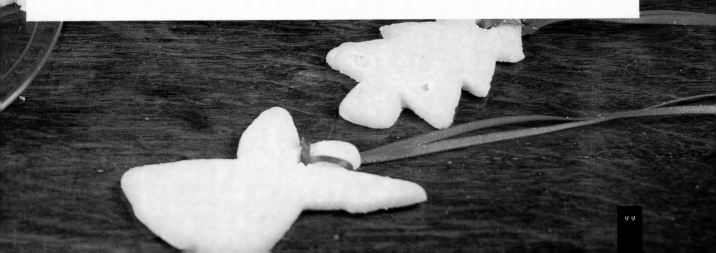

Bishop's Wine

BISHOP'S WINE was originally based on wassail, an early Saxon drink of hot ale flavored with sugar and spices, and topped with the pulp of roasted apples.

In Holland, children receive their Christmas presents on the feast of St. Nicholas in early December. Presents, which are all signed by St. Nicholas, are put in a basket and left on the doorstep. This is brought in and presents are

TO SERVE 8 PEOPLE YOU WILL NEED

2 bottles red wine

1 orange stuck with cloves

Peel of 1 lemon, 1 cinnamon stick

¾ cup/6oz (175g) sugar

METHOD

✳ *The day before you are planning to drink the bishop's wine, pour the red wine into a pot. Leave the orange stuck with cloves to marinade in it.*

✳ *The following day, simmer the wine together with the orange, lemon peel, cinnamon stick and sugar for about 30 minutes. Make sure it does not get to boiling point. Serve hot.*

distributed while members of the family eat sweet pastries and drink hot chocolate or bishop's wine.

Our recipe for bishop's wine is a simplified version of the better-known spiced mulled wine.

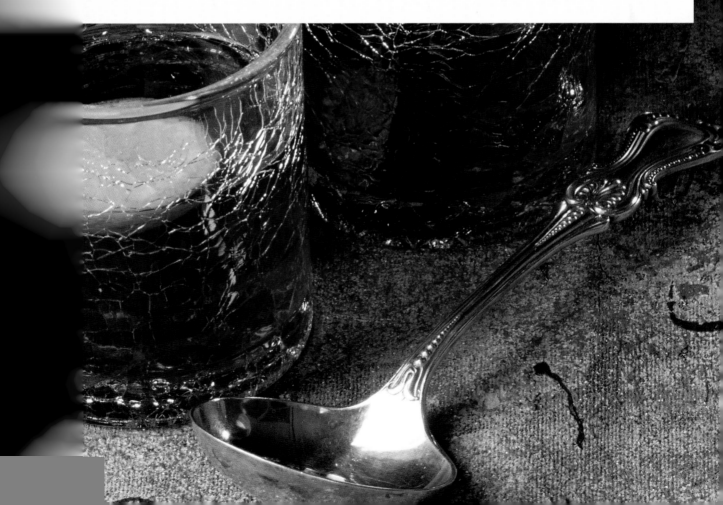

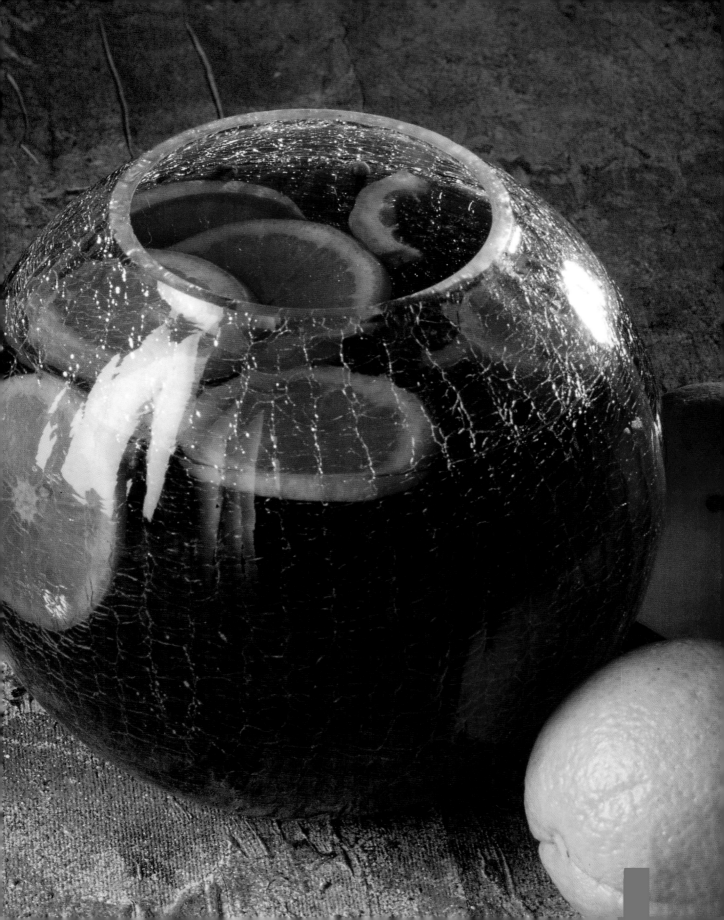

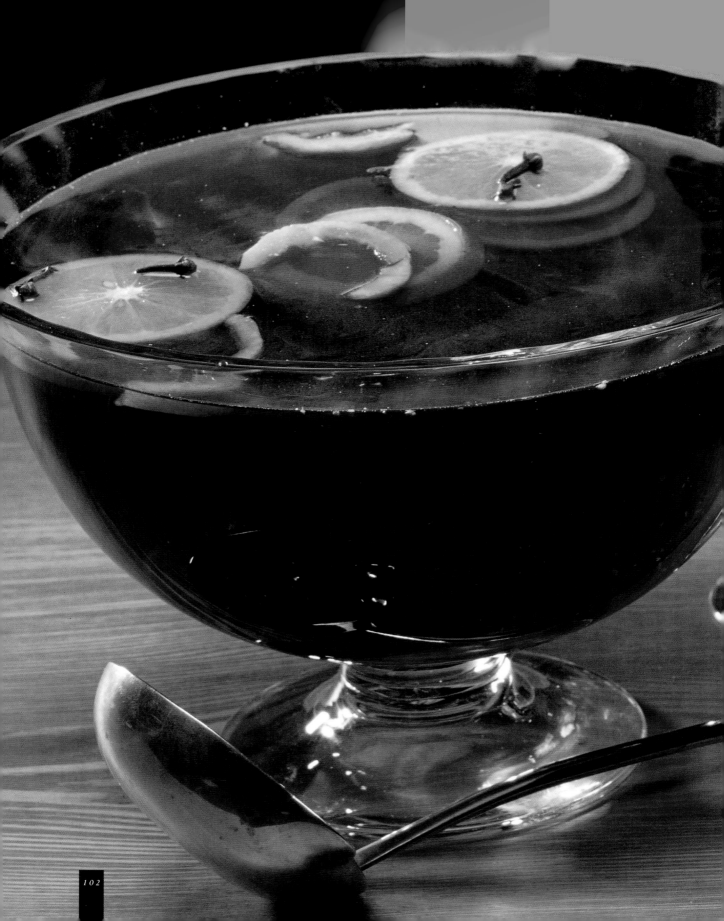

Mulled Wine

MULLED WINE can be kept in a large pot on the stove throughout the entire Christmas period. Not only will its sweet, spicy aromatic smell pervade the house in a most welcoming way, but it can be topped up frequently with more fruit, wine, sugar, and honey – plus an additional pot of hot Assam tea!

TO SERVE 18 PEOPLE YOU WILL NEED

4 oranges, Peel of 2 lemons

3 bottles full-bodied red wine

1 large teapot of strong black tea (preferably Assam)

6 tblsp honey, ½ cup/4oz (100g) sugar

3 cinnamon sticks, ½ whole nutmeg, grated

2 tsp cloves, 1 glass brandy

METHOD

❋ *Slice the oranges and peel the lemons. Put these in a saucepan with the 3 bottles of wine, strong black tea, honey, sugar, brandy, cloves, cinnamon and nutmeg.*

❋ *Heat gently, at simmering point, for about 30 minutes. The sweetness of the wine can be adjusted with honey and sugar as desired. Be careful not to boil the mixture or the alcohol will evaporate.*

❋ *The mulled wine can be prepared in advance and gently re-heated when required. Serve in warmed wine glasses, or decorative mugs with handles.*

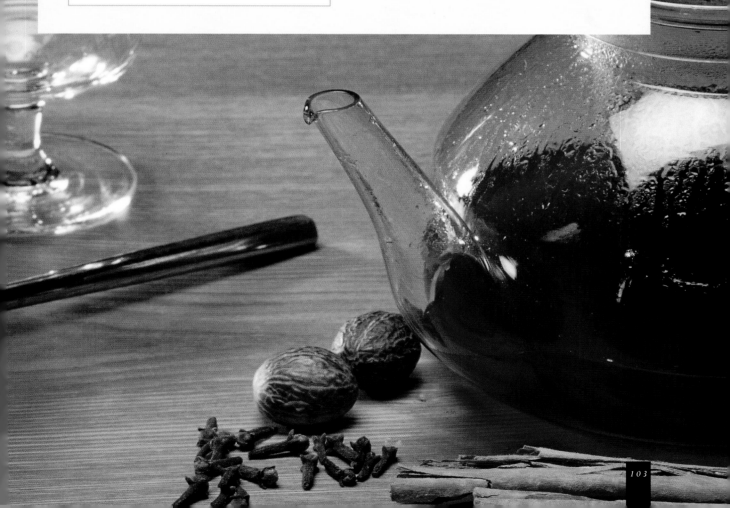

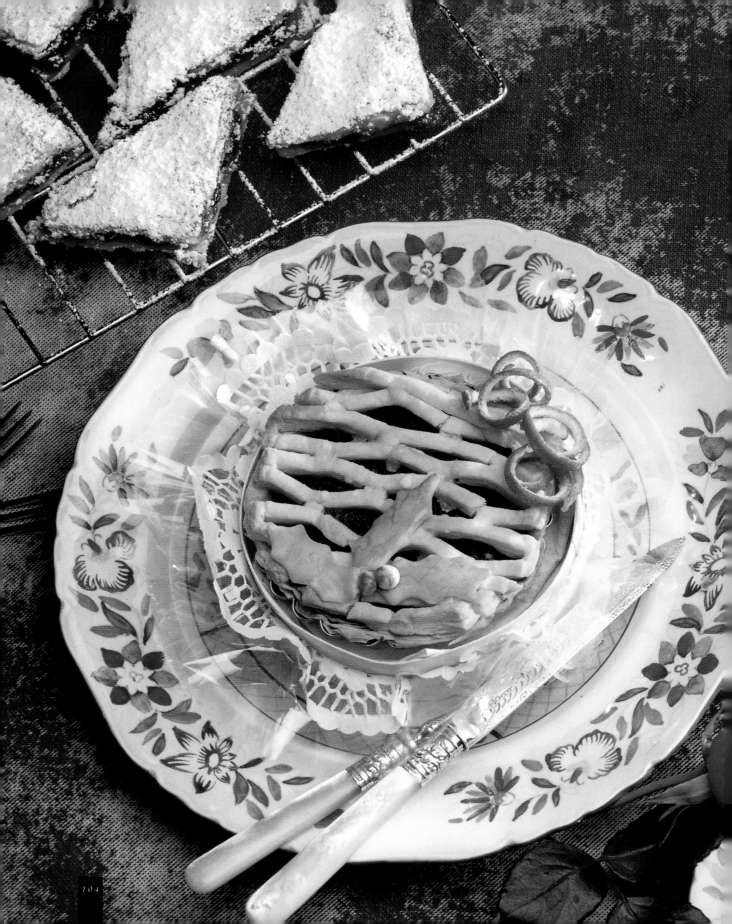

Mince Pies

MINCEMEAT, as we know it today, derives from a medieval English meat pie recipe which contained layers of meat and game interspersed with raisins, dates, sugar, prunes and ginger, surrounded by walls of pastry. Mince pies were standard Christmas fare by the seventeenth century, with fruit used in equal quantities to meat. In the nineteenth century, meat was omitted altogether and only the addition of suet reminds us of the original recipe. In the USA however, meat is still sometimes included.

Mincemeat is usually made between early October and mid-December, and put to store in a cool place. This recipe makes about 6lb (3kg) mincemeat.

MINCEMEAT

YOU WILL NEED 3 large sharp apples,
Rind and juice of 3 lemons and 3 oranges
½ cup/2oz (50g) blanched almonds or hazelnuts,
½ cup/2oz (50g) walnuts,
½ cup/4oz (100g) glacé/candied cherries,
½ cup/4oz (100g) figs or dates,
2 cups/12oz (350g) stoneless raisins,
2 cups/12oz (350g) currants,
½ cup/4oz (100g) mixed candied peel, 3 cups/12oz (350g) suet
(vegetarians can substitute shredded Vegetable Suenut)
2 cups/12oz (350g) sultanas, ½ tsp grated nutmeg,
½ tsp cinnamon, ½ tsp mace, ½ tsp ground cloves,
1½ cups/12oz (350g) sugar, 2 tblsp orange preserve,
¼ cup/6fl.oz (175ml) brandy or rum

✽ Bake the apples in a preheated oven at 180°C/350°F/Gas mark 4 for about 35-40 minutes until soft. Remove the skin from the apples and add the pulp to the rind and juice of the oranges and lemons.

✽ Chop the walnuts and almonds (or hazelnuts) coarsely. Do the same with the cherries and figs (or dates).

✽ Mix all the ingredients together, adding the brandy last. Leave for a few hours before spooning into clean jars. Cover with wax discs and seal. Store for at least a fortnight before using the mincemeat in recipes.

MINCE PIES

YOU WILL NEED ½ cup/3oz (75g) cream cheese,
½ cup/3oz (75g) butter,
3 cups/12oz (350g) plain flour, Pinch salt,
Cold water, Icing/confectioner's sugar,
A little milk, 1lb (450g) mincemeat

✽ Preheat the oven to 200°C/400°F/Gas mark 6. Blend together the cream cheese and the butter.

✽ Stir in the flour, sugar and salt. Add a small amount of cold water to bind the pastry. Leave it in the refrigerator for 30 minutes, wrapped in polythene.

✽ Grease small round pastry tins. Roll out the pastry, cut into small rounds and place in the tins. Fill with mincemeat. Dampen the edges with milk, cover with a second round of pastry for a lid, and pinch the edges together.

✽ Brush the tops of the pies with milk. Bake for about 25 minutes, then sprinkle the pies with icing (confectioner's) sugar.

✽ Mince pies can also be made in different shapes. We made a lattice tart, decorated with holly shapes made from rolled icing sugar; triangles and squares were made in a swiss roll tin (jelly roll pan).

Stollen Cake and Bread

THROUGHOUT EUROPE, traditional cakes and pastries are made at Christmas. Perhaps the best known of these is the German *Christstollen,* which is a rich fruit loaf, filled with dried fruit, nuts, candied cherries and peel. Symbolically, its traditional oval shape represents the baby Jesus wrapped in swaddling clothes.

Serve it on Christmas Eve with a glass of mulled wine, cider or ale. Stollen freezes well. It is delicious lightly toasted and served with butter. The loaves may be stuffed with marzipan.

FOR 2 STOLLEN (2 LOAVES) YOU WILL NEED

¾ cup/4oz (100g) seedless raisins

¾ cup/4oz (100g) currants

¾ cup/4oz (100g) mixed candied citrus peel

½ cup/3oz (75g) stoned dates

½ cup/3oz (75g) glacé/candied cherries, cut in half

½ cup/3oz (75g) blanched almonds or walnuts

3 tblsp lukewarm water, 1oz (25g) fresh yeast

1lb (450g) strong white flour,

⅞ cup/7fl.oz (210ml) warm milk, ½ tsp salt, 2 eggs

2 tsp finely grated fresh lemon rind/orange peel

¾ cup/6oz (175g) unsalted butter, in small pieces

½ cup/4oz (100g) melted unsalted butter

¾ cup/6oz (175g) sugar, Pinch ground mace

Pinch ground cinnamon

¼ cup/1oz (25g) icing/confectioner's sugar for dusting

Optional: 6oz (175g) marzipan

METHOD

❋ Warm the milk. Blend the yeast with the warm milk, ⅛ cup/1oz (25g) of sugar and 1 cup/4oz (100g) sifted flour. Set aside in a warm place until bubbly.

❋ Mix the raisins, currants, candied peel, dates, almonds and cherries in a bowl.

❋ Sift the remaining flour into a large bowl, together with the salt, mace and cinnamon. Blend the milk and yeast with the remaining sugar, and stir in. Add the grated lemon or orange rind.

❋ Beat the eggs. With a wooden spoon, cream together the small pieces of butter and eggs. Then slowly mix this into the flour, blending thoroughly. Now work in the mixture of fruits and nuts as evenly as possible. Divide the dough into two.

❋ Leave the bowl of dough in a warm place, covered with a towel or saran wrap, until the dough has doubled in size (1-2 hours). Knead the dough again briefly, knocking all the air out of it. Roll out the dough and shape into an oblong.

❋ If you wish to stuff one or both of the loaves with marzipan, now is the time to do it. Place the marzipan in the center of the dough in a sausage shape, which does not touch the edges.

❋ Put both loaves on a greased cookie sheet, cover and leave to rise again in a warm place until they have doubled in size (about 1½ hours). Brush both loaves with the melted butter and bake in at 190°C/ 375°F /Gas mark 5 for 35-40 minutes.

❋ Allow the loaves to cool for 5 minutes before removing to a wire rack. Once cool, dust with the sifted icing (confectioner's) sugar.

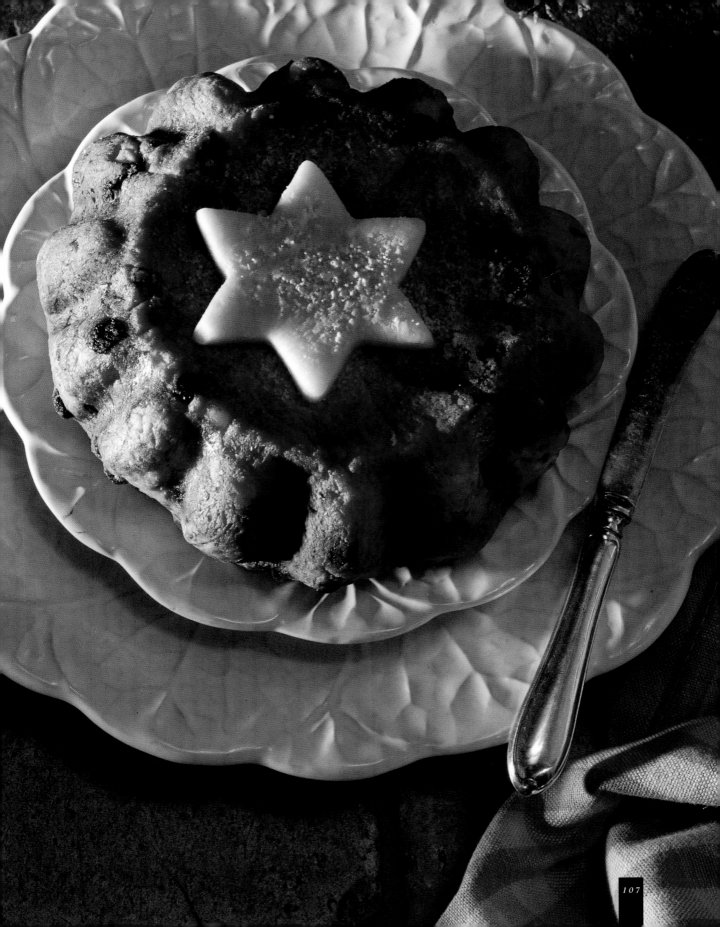

Nut Roast with Cranberry Sauce

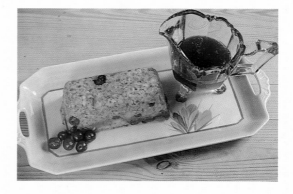

YOU WILL NEED

½ cup/4oz (100g) plus ¼ cup/2oz (50g) butter

2 medium-sized onions, finely chopped

2 garlic cloves, crushed

2 small eating apples, peeled and diced

5 sticks celery, finely chopped

1½ cups/8oz (225g) finely chopped brazil nuts

1½ cups/8oz (225g) toasted and chopped
ground cashew nuts

1 cup/4oz (100g) rolled oats

1 cup/4oz (100g) cooked and mashed parsnip

2 tblsp chopped parsley, 1 tsp fresh sage

½ tsp dried oregano, ½ tsp ground ginger

½ tsp cumin, Stock or white wine to taste

Salt and pepper

METHOD

✳ Grease a paper-lined 2lb (1kg) loaf tin. Melt the
smaller quantity of butter in a saucepan, add the
onions and cook gently for about 10 minutes
until onions are softened. Add the crushed garlic,
together with the apple and celery. Cook briefly
for another minute.

✳ Mix together brazil and cashew nuts, oats, parsnips,
parsley, larger quantity of butter, and white wine or
stock. Add the sage, oregano, ginger and cumin, and
mix thoroughly. Season generously with salt and
pepper to taste.

✳ Press half the mixture into the tin. Spread the
chestnut stuffing evenly over it. Press down well. Top
this with the remaining half of the nut mixture.
Bake in a moderate oven at 190°C /375°F /Gas
mark 5 for 45 minutes to an hour, until golden
brown. Serve sliced, with cranberry sauce.

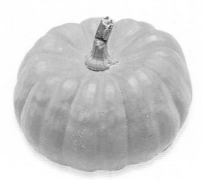

Prune, Apricot, And Walnut Stuffing

TURKEY WAS INTRODUCED by the British to New England in the form of an improved breed of the Mexican turkey, bred in Norfolk, the main turkey-rearing area in Britain.

In the eighteenth century, turkey was used in the famous Yorkshire Christmas pies, where birds were stuffed one inside the other. A goose, which was stuffed with a fowl, into which was stuffed a partridge, stuffed with a pigeon, was inserted into a boned turkey! Our somewhat simpler stuffing is based on a Breton recipe, with Persian influences.

YOU WILL NEED
TO STUFF A 10LB (5KG) TURKEY

2 finely chopped onions, 4 tblsp butter, 1½lb (675g) pork

3 rashers lean unsmoked bacon, 2 heaped tblsp parsley

3 heaped tblsp breadcrumbs

1 tsp each cumin and cinnamon

½ tsp each of ground cloves and nutmeg

1lb (450g) dried apricots, soaked and chopped

1lb (450g) prunes, soaked in tea, stoned and chopped

¾ cup/4oz (100g) broken walnuts,

6oz (175g) field mushrooms

Salt, and freshly-ground black pepper to taste

FOR ROASTING THE BIRD:

½ cup/4oz (100g) butter

SAUCE:

1 glass brandy or port

1¼ cups/½pt (300ml) double (heavy) cream

METHOD

❋ To make the stuffing, sauté the onions in butter until soft, together with the bacon and diced pork. Add the mushrooms and cook gently. Mix together with all the other ingredients. Season to taste with salt and pepper.

❋ Rub the bird lavishly all over with the butter, particularly over the breast. Spoon the stuffing into the body cavity. Lay the bird on one side in a roasting tin, covered with tin foil. Cook at 170°C /325°F /Gas mark 3 for 3-4 hours, according to the weight of the bird. Be sure to turn it on to its other side halfway through the cooking process, and keep it covered with foil. Baste with butter during cooking. When the bird is nearly cooked, remove the foil and turn the bird on to its back to ensure an even color.

❋ Transfer the bird to a warm serving dish and leave it to stand for five minutes before carving.

❋ To make the sauce, skim off the surplus fat from the pan juices and throw it away. Boil up the juices with a glass of brandy or port. Add the cream and season.

❋ Alternatively, form the stuffing mixture into balls, place on a greased cookie sheet, and bake separately at 190°C /375°F /Gas mark 5 for 40 minutes.

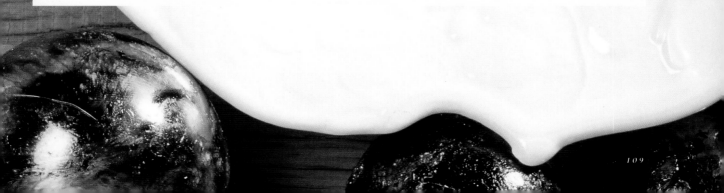

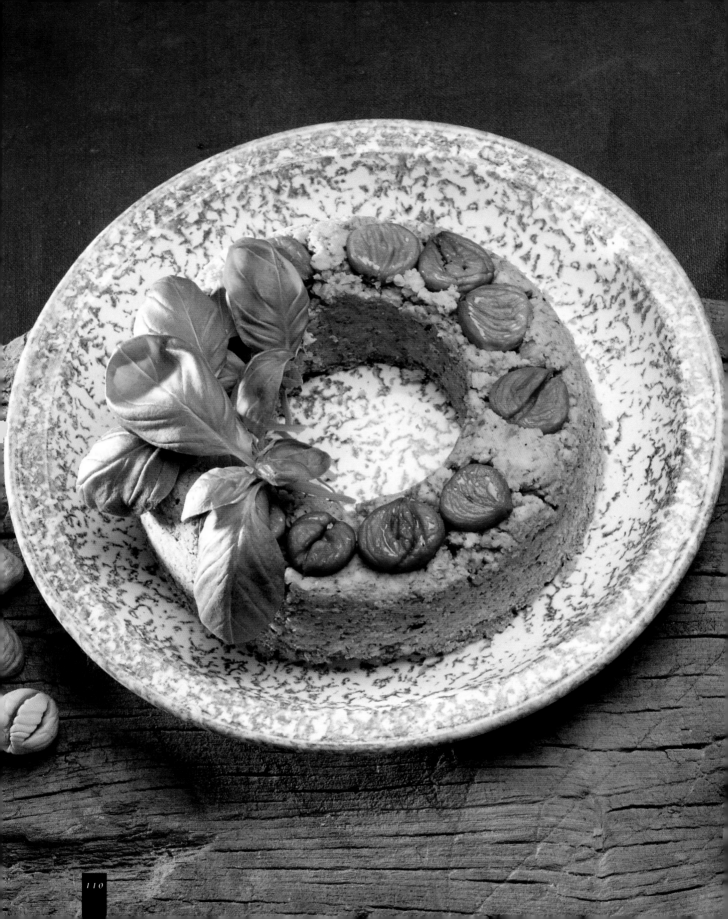

Chestnut Stuffing

IN BRITAIN DURING the cold days leading up to Christmas, many a city street is enlivened by the sight of a hot charcoal burner emitting the warm sweet smell of roasting chestnuts.

Chestnuts can be eaten raw, baked as bread (popular in the Mediterranean), or made into soup. They also make a delicious pudding with spices and almonds, or simply served as marrons glacés, another Christmas treat. Our chestnut stuffing can be served with meat or vegetarian dishes.

YOU WILL NEED

2 cups/8oz (225g) whole chestnuts

1 cup/2oz (50g) wholemeal breadcrumbs

Rind and juice of half a lemon

1 lightly beaten egg

½ tsp fresh grated nutmeg

3 tblsp fresh chopped basil leaves

METHOD

❋ Cook the chestnuts by boiling whole in their skins for about half an hour. Peel away the skin. Reserve a few whole chestnuts for the bottom of the mold, and for decoration, and mash the rest. (You can also use dried or canned chestnuts, or chestnut purée for this recipe.)

❋ To make the stuffing, mix together the mashed chestnuts, egg, nutmeg, breadcrumbs, lemon rind, lemon juice and basil.

❋ Grease a ring mold, and scatter a few whole nuts in the bottom. Press the stuffing mixture in. Bake at 190°C /375°F /Gas mark 5 for 40 minutes.

❋ Turn out of the mold and decorate with the reserved chestnuts. Serve with a garnish of basil.

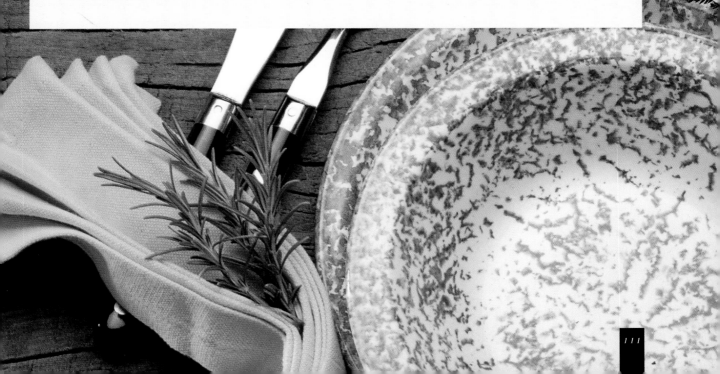

Christmas Cake

TRADITIONAL CHRISTMAS CAKE recipes vary from country to country. Britain has a very rich, heavy fruit cake, with or without marzipan and royal icing; Italy has a much lighter, airier fruit cake called *pannetone*. The French serve a chocolate log, *bûche de Noel*, and the Germans enjoy *Christstollen*, a rich fruit loaf. In the USA, fruit cakes are made without marzipan and royal icing.

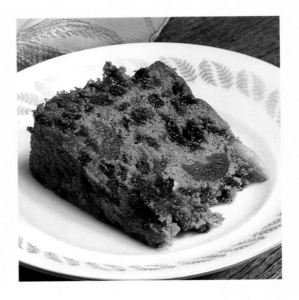

RICH FRUIT CAKE

2½ cups/1lb (450g) sultanas, 1¼ cups/8oz (225g) currants

1¼ cups/8oz (225g) stoned dates,

1 cup/5oz (150g) seedless raisins

½ cup/2oz (50g) candied peel, shredded, ½ cup/2oz (50g) glacé cherries, halved (candied cherries),

½ cup/2oz (50g) chopped walnuts,

½ cup/2oz (50g) blanched almonds, chopped

Grated rind of 1 orange, Grated rind of 1 lemon,

⅔ cup/¼pt (150ml) brandy or rum (or orange juice),

1 tsp cinnamon, 1 tsp grated nutmeg,

1 tsp allspice, 1 tsp ground cloves, Pinch of salt

1½ cups/12oz (350g) butter, 1½ cups/12oz (350g) brown sugar

2 tblsp black treacle, 6 eggs, 4 cups/1lb (450g) plain flour,

Optional: marzipan and royal icing

❋ *Make the cake about a month before eating, to give time for the flavor to mature.*

❋ *The night before, put the mixed fruit, candied peel, orange and lemon rind and nuts in a bowl, and pour on the brandy and rum. Cover the bowl.*

❋ *The following day, pre-heat the oven to 140°C/ 275°F / Gas mark 1. Cream together the butter and sugar.*

❋ *Beat the eggs separately. Mix carefully into the butter and sugar mixture a little at a time, so that it does not curdle.*

❋ *Sift the flour into another bowl. Mix in the spices. Gradually fold the flour mixture into the eggs, butter and sugar, blending well. Do not beat. Lift the dried fruit and nut mixture out of the brandy with a spatula and add to the cake mixture. Finally, add the treacle and the brandy.*

❋ *Transfer to a greased cake tin, cover with a double piece of greaseproof paper, and bake for 5-6 hours. After 5 hours, check to see if the cake is cooked by inserting a fine skewer or a knitting needle in the centre. If it is cooked, the skewer will come out clean.*

❋ *Remove the cake from the oven and let it cool in the tin for 30 minutes before turning on to a wire rack. Wrap in double greaseproof paper. Feed periodically with brandy or rum (or orange juice) by pouring through small holes pierced in the cake.*

❋ *Serve the cake as it is, or cover with marzipan and icing shortly before Christmas.*

MARZIPAN

1½ cups/6oz (175g) icing sugar (confectioner's sugar)

¾ cup/6oz (175g) caster sugar (granulated sugar)

3 cups/12oz (350g) ground almonds

2 eggs, 1-2 tblsp lemon juice, 1 tblsp brandy, 6 drops vanilla essence, 6 drops almond essence

✳ *Sift both types of sugar into a bowl. Mix in the ground almonds.*

✳ *Beat the eggs together with 1 tablespoonful of the lemon juice, the brandy, vanilla and almond essences. Add slowly to the dry ingredients, working in well to make a smooth paste. Add more lemon juice if required.*

✳ *Divide into two portions of two-thirds and one-third each. Use the larger portion of marzipan to cover the sides of the cake, and the smaller portion for the top. Now ice with royal icing.*

ROYAL ICING

4½ cups/1½lb (675g) icing sugar (confectioner's sugar)

4 egg whites, 2 tsp lemon juice

1 tsp rosewater, 1 tsp glycerine

✳ *Whisk the egg whites until frothy. Slowly sift in the sugar, mixing with a wooden spoon. Beating well, gradually add small amounts of the lemon juice, rosewater and glycerine (which prevent the icing from hardening). Keep beating until the icing stands up in stiff peaks.*

✳ *Cover with a damp cloth and leave for up to two hours, before icing the cake.*

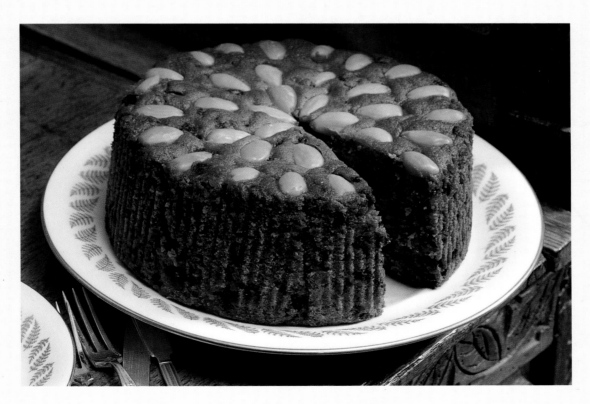

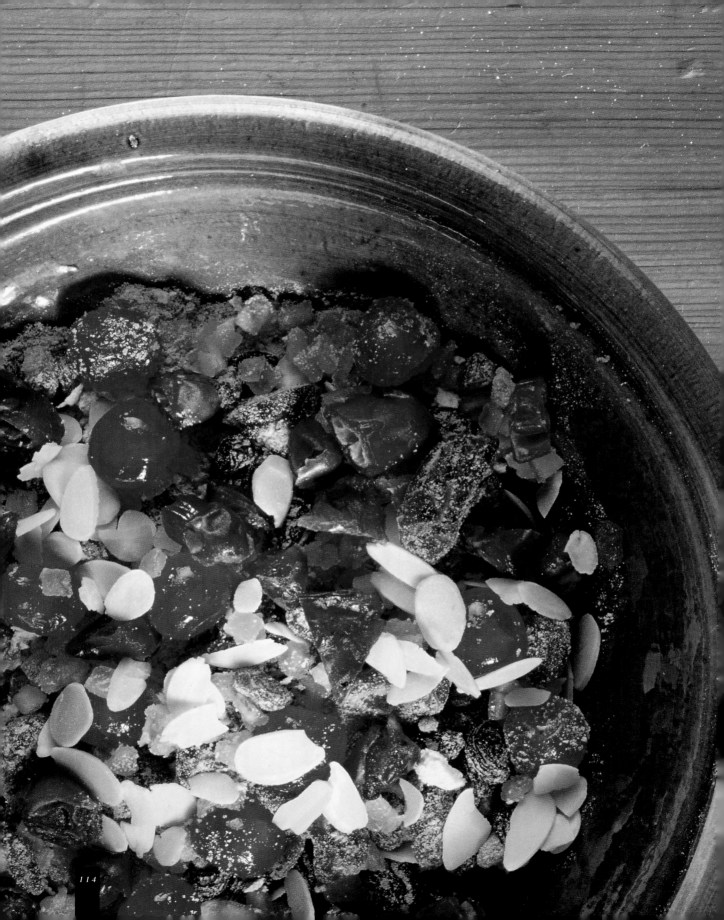

Plum Pudding

PLUM PUDDING (or Christmas pudding) seems quintessentially English, but was originally a Greek dish. Plum pudding in fact rarely contains plums, and developed from the Christmas porridge or broth which was popular in the sixteenth century. It was called by various names such as plum pottage, plum broth or Christmas pottage, and was eaten as a first course. This tradition is echoed in Scandinavian countries today, where a dish of sweetened rice-grain porridge is eaten as a first course, to line the stomach before the richer second courses.

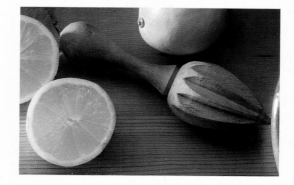

The original recipe contained chunks of beef cooked in wine with onions, herbs, bread and aromatic spices such as cloves, mace and cinnamon. Raisins and currants were also essential ingredients and in Tudor times, prunes (dried plums) were added. In the seventeenth century, plum pudding was banished by the Puritans in Britain, only to re-emerge in the reign of Charles II.

Although plum broth was predominant in the eighteenth century, by the nineteenth century a more solid plum pudding had become popular. It was, however, only in 1836 that the plum pudding became exclusively associated with Christmas and re-named the Christmas pudding. By the early nineteenth century, meat was no longer included.

Christmas pudding displaced Twelfth Night cake in popularity, and also inherited from it the tradition of including charms in the mixture: a silver threepenny piece for good fortune, a thimble for a spinster, a button for a bachelor. A ring foretold a wedding and a tiny horseshoe brought good luck.

Traditionally, the pudding is made on Stir-up Sunday, which is the Sunday before Advent. This gives it time to mature. Every member of the family should participate in the ritual of stirring the pudding from east to west, in honor of the Three Kings, and making a silent wish for good fortune in the coming year.

Christmas Plum Pudding

FOR TWO PUDDINGS YOU WILL NEED

1¼ cups/8oz (225g) currants

1¼ cups/8oz (225g) chopped sultanas

1¼ cups/8oz (225g) seedless chopped raisins

¾ cup/4oz (100g) stoned, chopped dates

¾ cup/4oz (100g) chopped dried figs

½ cup/4oz (100g) glacé cherries

¾ cup/4oz (100g) mixed peel, chopped

1 cup/4oz (100g) blanched, slivered almonds

4 cups/8oz (225g) fresh white breadcrumbs

1 cups/8oz (225g) soft brown sugar
(firmly packed light and dark brown sugar)

2 cups/8oz (225g) prepared shredded suet
(or shredded Vegetable Suenut)

Finely grated rind and juice of one orange

Finely grated rind and juice of one lemon

2 cups/8oz (225g) plain flour , Pinch salt

1 level tsp ground mace,

1 level tsp ground cinnamon

1 level tsp mixed spice

4 large eggs, beaten

1¼cups/½pt (300ml) sweet brown ale

⅔ cup/¼pt (150ml) stout

6 tblsp dark rum or brandy

TO SERVE

3 tblsp brandy, heated and a sprig of holly

METHOD

✳ It takes two days to prepare plum puddings. On the first day, sift the flour into a large mixing bowl with the spices and salt. Add the suet, breadcrumbs and sugar. Gradually mix in all the diced dried fruit and nuts, together with the orange and lemon rinds and grated apple.

✳ In a separate bowl, beat the eggs together with the sweet brown ale, stout and rum or brandy. Stir the liquid slowly into the dry mixture, making sure that it binds evenly. (At this point you can add silver charms, if you wish.) Cover and leave to stand overnight to allow the flavors to develop.

✳ On the second day, grease two 2pt (1 liter) pudding basins. Divide the pudding mixture into two and distribute it between the two basins. Pack the mixture in firmly and cover the tops of the basins with buttered greaseproof paper or aluminum foil, leaving enough space for the pudding to rise.

✳ Cover the top with a clean piece of linen or a folded tea towel. Tie securely with a piece of string. Fill a very large pan with enough boiling water to come halfway up the pudding basins. Place the basins in the pan and steam for 8 hours. Make sure that the water does not boil away.

✳ Store in a cool, dry place if prepared before Christmas. On Christmas Day, the dish should be steamed again for a further three hours until thoroughly heated through. Before serving, decorate with a sprig of holly. Pour over the brandy, flame and serve with brandy butter or clotted cream.

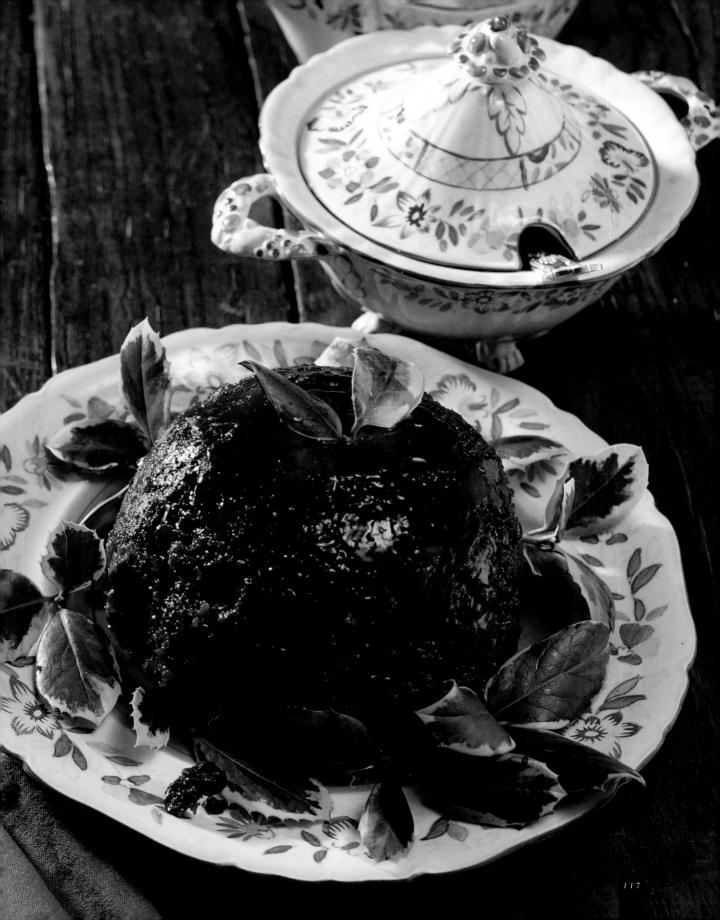

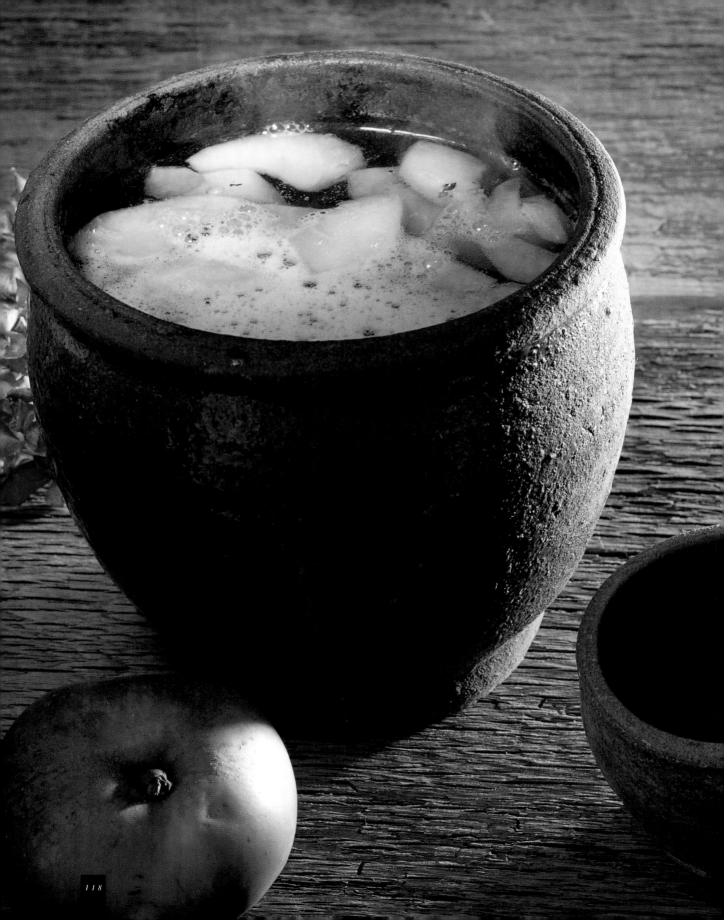

Wassail

THE DRINKING OF WASSAIL, hot spiced ale with apple foam on top, goes back to Anglo-Saxon times. In Britain the custom of "wassailing" fruit orchards still persists today. Libations of cider or ale are poured on to the roots of apple or plum trees with great ceremony to ensure that the following year's crop of fruit will be good.

Traditionally the apple foam topping, known as "lamb's wool," was made by heating apples, which then exploded open on contact with the hot ale. This warming, festive drink was much enjoyed by the diarist Samuel Pepys and his contemporaries in the seventeenth century.

On New Year's Eve, family and friends would gather together to drink from a bowl of wassail. The head of the family would drink first, calling out "Waes hael" (an old Saxon phrase meaning "Good health" from which the word "wassail" comes). Each person declared the same toast as they drank, wishing good health and happiness to all present. Sometimes the wassail bowl was decorated with sprigs of holly, bells and ribbons and taken from house to house. It was thought to bring good fortune to those who drank from it.

YOU WILL NEED

18 cups/6pt (3.6 litres) brown ale

2 cups/1lb (450g) soft brown sugar
(firmly packed light and dark brown sugar)

6 cooking apples, 1 stick cinnamon

10 cardamom pods, cracked

1 tsp grated fresh nutmeg, 1 tsp ground ginger

1¼ cups/½pt (300ml) Calvados or sweet white wine

METHOD

✳ *Core and peel the apples, and bake at 140°C/ 275°F /Gas mark 1 until soft. Cut the apples into small pieces and keep warm.*

✳ *While the apples are cooking, heat the ale gently with the sugar, spices and Calvados, without letting it boil. Leave to infuse on a warm stove for half an hour.*

✳ *Remove the cardamom pods and cinnamon. Pour into an earthenware bowl and top with the warm apple pieces.*

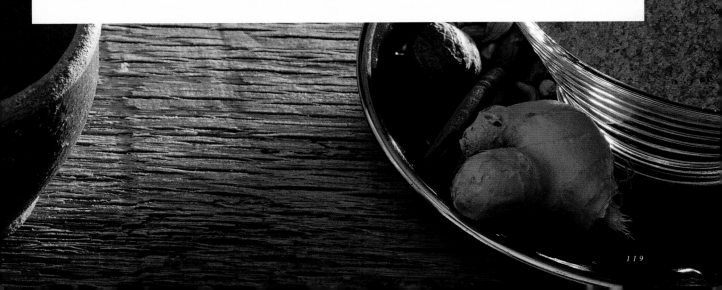

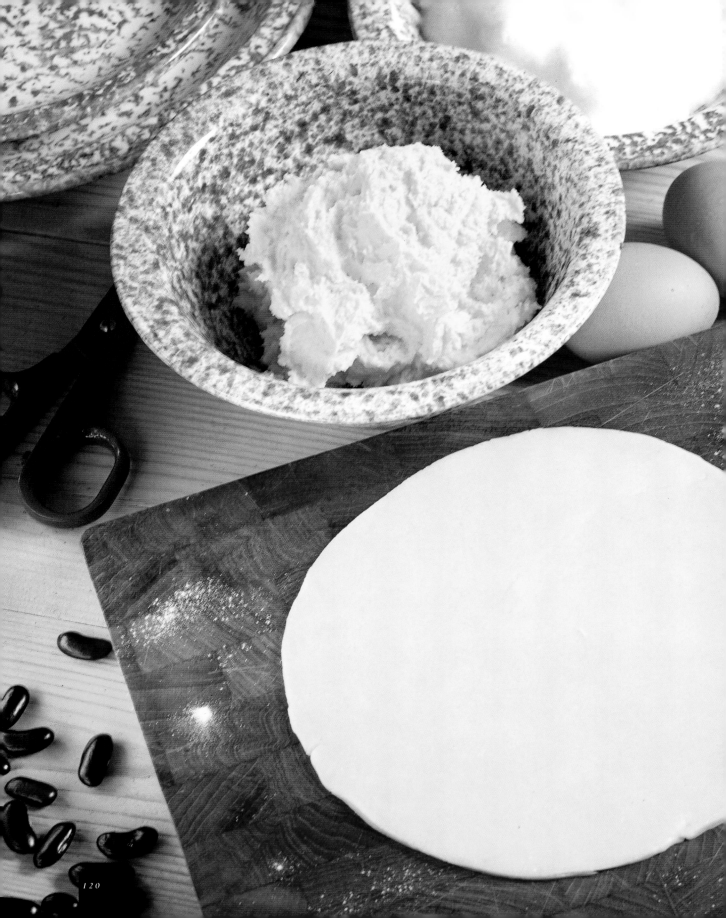

Twelfth Night Cake

TWELFTH NIGHT CAKE (which is actually more like a pie) is eaten on Epiphany, the twelfth night after Christmas, when festivities draw to a close and the tree and decorations are taken down.

The cake was traditionally decorated with a golden crown to symbolize the Three Kings' visit to baby Jesus in Bethlehem on the twelfth night after his birth. Modern cakes may have small figures of the Three Kings on top.

The tradition of including charms in the Christmas pudding owes its origin to the custom of hiding a bean and a pea inside the Twelfth Night cake. Traditionally, Twelfth Night was a night of revelry and excess, and whoever found the bean was crowned the King of the revels. The pea was awarded to the lady of his choice, who became Queen for the evening. Twelfth Night cake became less popular in the 1850s, when Christmas pudding took over as the universal Christmas sweet dish.

GALETTE DES ROIS

The tradition of Twelfth Night cake is still maintained in France, where it is called *galette des rois* (Three Kings cake). The bean is often replaced by a china bean or porcelain baby Jesus, or a metal charm. Most cakes are made to a Parisian recipe, with flaky pastry, although there are numerous regional differences.

Shops in France begin selling the cakes just after New Year's Day. They come complete with a gilded cardboard crown, to be worn by whoever finds the bean or charm. French families often invite friends to dinner on Twelfth Night, and *galette des rois* will be served after the meal.

In some places it has become customary for the lucky person who finds the charm (and who therefore becomes the King) to buy or make the cake (and often to buy the champagne as well) for the following year's celebrations.

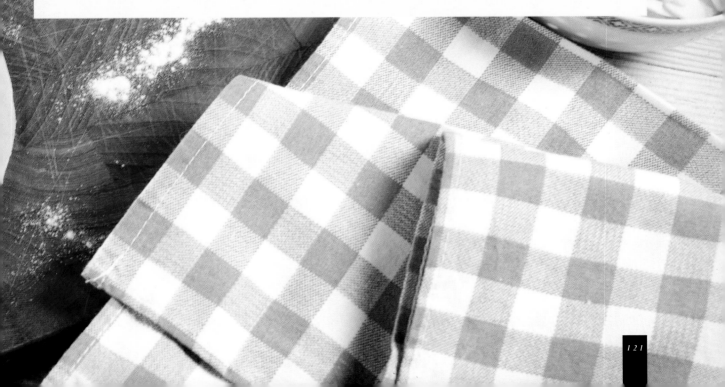

Twelfth Night Cake "Galette des Rois"

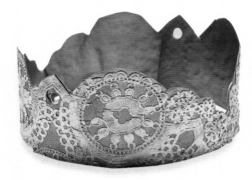

YOU WILL NEED

1lb (450g) puff pastry or sweet shortcrust pastry

¾ cup/6oz (175g) unsalted butter

¾ cup/6oz (175g) caster sugar (granulated sugar)

4 egg yolks, 4 egg whites, stiffly beaten

4 tsp Grand Marnier, brandy or kirsch

1½ cups/6oz (175g) fresh ground almonds

6 drops vanilla essence

Optional: I dried bean and I dried pea

Icing sugar (confectioner's sugar)

METHOD

✷ Pre-heat the oven to 190°C /375°F /Gas mark 5. Cream together the butter and sugar until fluffy. Blend together three egg yolks with the ground almonds, vanilla essence and liqueur.

✷ Beat the four egg whites until stiff.

✷ Divide the pastry in two and roll into two equally-shaped rounds of dough. Grease a baking tin and place one round in it.

✷ Now fold in the egg whites into the egg yolk, butter and sugar mixture, adding in the dried bean and pea if required.

✷ Spoon the mixture into the baking tin. Beat the remaining egg yolk and paint the pastry margin with it. Place the second round of dough on top and pinch the two edges together. Carefully cut a star out of spare pastry, paint with beaten egg, and put on top. Paint the pastry lid with beaten egg.

✷ Bake for 35-40 minutes until the pastry is browned. Let the cake cool, and then sprinkle sifted icing sugar on top. Decorate with a gold cardboard crown or small figurines of the Three Kings.

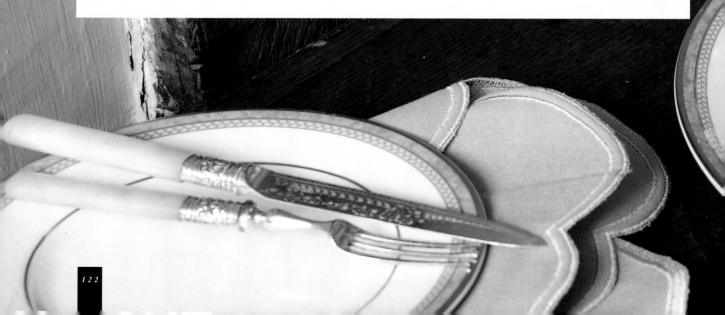

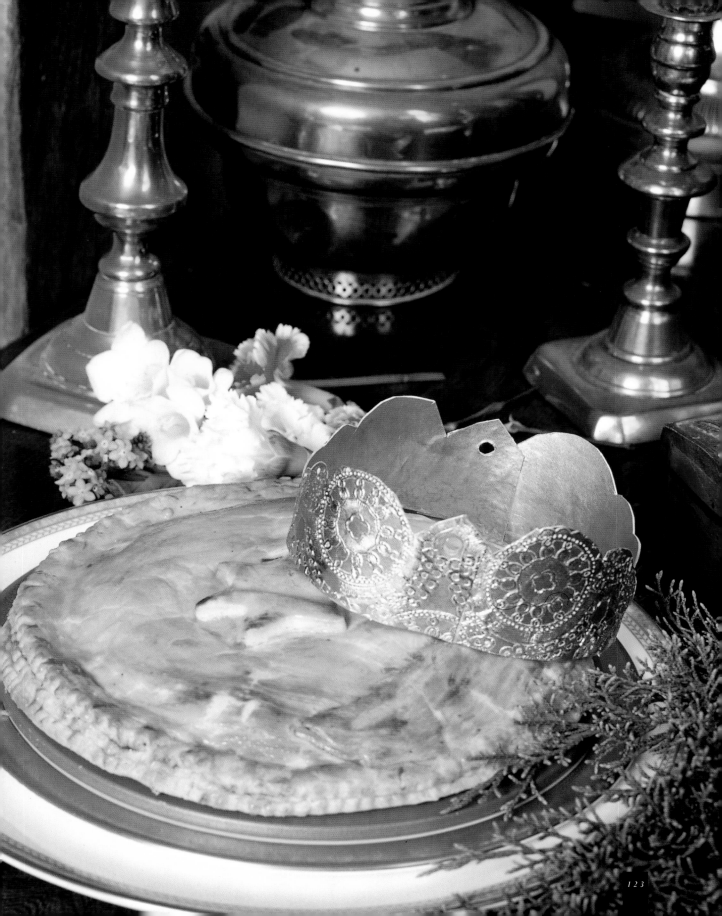

ACKNOWLEDGEMENTS

I would like to thank the following people, who helped in various ways during the writing of this book. Firstly, I would like to thank Judith Allan for her extensive research and imaginative contribution to the cookery section of the book. I could not have completed the project without her! I would especially like to acknowledge the contributions of all my friends who offered their own creative ideas, especially Chris Ackerman, Angelica Bradley, Eileen Lawless, Glynis Maine, Sarah Moreland, Sue Wales and Diana Wells. Thanks also to Julia Hull for her enthusiasm, suggestions and excellent culinary advice; Celia and Brian Wright for lending material, especially early cookery books; Lalita du Perron for help and encouragement; Jill Purce for helpful suggestions and use of her extensive library; Cara Denman for guidance; Hetty MacLise and Alan Hodgson for encouragement and tasting/testing recipes. Last but not least, I would like to thank my husband Alec and my ten-year-old daughter Natasha. Natasha, in particular, proved to be an invaluable accomplice throughout, not only by coming up with innovative, decorative ideas but also by helping to put them into practice!

BIBLIOGRAPHY

The Illustrated Encyclopedia of Essential Oils by Julia Lawless (Element, 1995)

The Complete Illustrated Guide to Aromatherapy by Julia Lawless (Element, 1997)

Aromatherapy and the Mind by Julia Lawless (Thorsons, 1994)

Complete Book of Herbs by Geraldine Holt (BCA, 1991)

The Creative Book of Flower Fragrance by Joanna Sheen (Salamander, 1992)

Aromatics by Angela Flanders (Mitchell Beazley, 1995)

Aromatic Gifts by Stephanie Donaldson (New Holland, 1995)

Blue Ribbon Book of Herb and Spice Cookery (Brooke Bond Oxo Ltd., 1971)

Herbs and Spices by Rosemary Hemphill (Penguin, 1966)

Spices, Salt and Aromatics in the English Kitchen by Elizabeth David (Penguin Books,1970)

A Feast of Scotland by Janet Warren (Lomond Books, 1979)

Christmas Fayre by Sara Paston-Williams (David & Charles, 1989)

Festivals, Family and Food by Diana Carey and Judy Large (Hawthorn Press, 1982)

Delia Smith's Christmas by Delia Smith (BBC Books, 1990)

The Christmas Cookbook by Nanette Newman (Hamlyn, 1984)

Christmas Cooking by Arabella Boxer (Hamlyn, 1988)

Good Housekeeping Cookery Club Cooking for Christmas by Maxine Clarke (Ebury Press, 1994)

Leith's Cookery Bible by Prue Leith and Caroline Waldegrave (Bloomsbury, 1991)

Two Fat Ladies by Jennifer Paterson & Clarissa Dickson Wright (Ebury Press, 1991)

Entertaining with Cranks by Kay Canter and Daphne Swann (Grafton Books, 1987)

Simply Delicious by Rose Elliot (Fletcher & Son, 1967)

Vegetarian Christmas by Rose Elliott (HarperCollins, 1992)

Vegetarian Kitchen by Sarah Brown (BBC, 1984)

The Feast of Christmas by Paul Levy (Kyle Cathie, 1992)

Festive Food and Party Pieces by Josceline Dimbleby (Woodhead-Faulkner for J. Sainsbury plc, 1982)

Country Living (December 1997)

Good Things by Jane Grigson (Penguin, 1973)

History of Food by Maguelonne Toussaint-Samat (Blackwell, 1994)

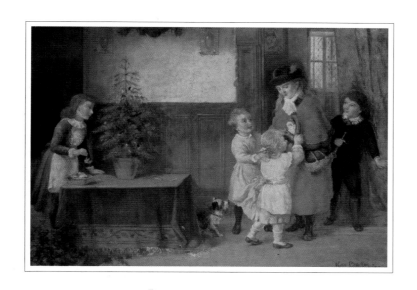

PICTURE CREDITS

The publishers are grateful to the following for permission
to reproduce copyright material

The Bridgeman Art Library: frontispiece, pp.11, 12,125

Fine Art Photographic Library: p 8